D1520913

CANCER FIGHT TO WIN

BREAST CANCER

SIX STEPS
to Achieve Remission

LAWRENCE W. DICKINS

CONTENTS

PROLOGUE

During our early years, when my brother and I were still quite young, our parents embarked on frequent travels, leaving us in the care of a young Peruvian woman in her early thirties. Over time, a deep affection blossomed between us and her, to the extent that in the years that followed, she became an integral part of our family, having even moved into our home. She transformed from being merely a caretaker to a cherished companion. As we pursued our education, she ventured into the corporate world as a secretary to an executive in the communications industry.

Then, one day, she vanished from our lives without a trace, replaced by a new caretaker. Our inquiries about her whereabouts were met with explanations that she needed to be away temporarily, attending to matters beyond our comprehension—things of an adult nature. Her return, though it felt like an eternity, marked a change. The essence of her presence seemed altered; she donned unfamiliar attire, and the warm embraces we once shared were now off-limits. Although we couldn't quite grasp the reasons, we obediently abided by the new boundaries.

As the years rolled on, we found ourselves being sent off to school in England. Yet, our homecomings for holidays remained a cherished tradition. The seaside visits, filled with joyous moments, still featured Helen's presence, though her lack of a bathing suit remained a puzzling oddity. Nevertheless, our affection for her endured, accepting these peculiarities for what they were.

As I matured, I grew curious about the transformation Helen had undergone—from a carefree girl to a more reserved and mature figure. Seeking answers, I turned to my mother, who finally unveiled the truth. She disclosed that Helen had undergone a double mastectomy, a decision she had struggled with and felt ashamed of. This revelation thrust me into the awareness of cancer, a devastating force that could reshape lives. This insight into the past took place during the 1960s, a time when radical mastectomies were the prevailing approach due to the nascent state of cancer treatment. The landscape of medical care was markedly different, with limited options and understanding.

Years later, in my early fifties, the impact of cancer hit home as I received my own diagnosis: Esophageal Cancer stage II. The perspective shift was profound, as I now found myself on the receiving end of what I had once encountered through Helen's experience.

However, the realm of cancer care has evolved significantly by now. Advanced imaging technologies and refined surgical tools have initiated a new era of treatments, rendering death from early-stage breast cancer a rarity.

While writing this very book, a call from my personal assistant interrupted my thoughts. She shared news of her own cancer diagnosis—an early-stage, Stage I Ductal Carcinoma in Situ in her left breast, detected during a routine checkup. Luckily, it had been caught at an early stage, and no lymph nodes were affected. Together, we went through the contents of this book, discussing the fundamental elements: understanding the nature of cancer, comprehending its progression, preparing for surgical intervention, and adopting optimal nutritional practices. Our conversations spanned various topics, and as the day of her surgery approached, she displayed remarkable calmness and clarity. The power of knowledge and understanding was evident, transforming fear into an informed approach to her impending journey.

Currently, she is doing well on her recovery path and eagerly anticipates embracing her role as a new grandparent. This narrative sums up the essence of this book—a beacon of information and guidance for those grappling with cancer. It intends to equip individuals with an understanding of the disease while providing practical guidelines to alleviate the emotional and mental burden that cancer patients inevitably face.

This book is dedicated to:

Helen and Lulu.

INTRODUCTION

In 2004, I was diagnosed with cancer.

In 2007, I was diagnosed with cancer.

I have been free of cancer ever since.

What changed?

This is what this book is about. The first-time doctors diagnosed my cancer, I went dutifully to the doctor and did all that he requested. I went into surgery and then into chemo and radiation.

Then I went back to my life with a renewed effort to pick up on lost time. I had been in treatment for nearly four months.

I went back to my old routine, traveling all over the world, eating whenever I had the opportunity or the time. Picking any type of sandwich and soft drink I could. Eating on the run. Sleeping on planes and then arriving directly to meetings. Come on, I was living the Jet-Set life of my dreams!

I worked for a TV Network as their agent distributing programs throughout Europe. I would attend TV Festivals in Cannes, France, Madrid, Spain, Prague, Czech Republic, and

Las Vegas, USA. Cocktail parties galore. Dinners every night entertaining clients attended by the various actresses and actors of the series. It was fun; it was trivial, and it was dangerous.

One day my body just said, "Stop, no more".

One fateful morning in June 2007, as I was traveling in Mexico, I decided to have a checkup, as I was sure that it was going to be routine. As I went for my results in the American and British Cowdry Hospital, I was told politely, and with certain discomfort, that my endoscopy had revealed a tumor, adenocarcinoma, in my esophagus. The good news was that it was at an early stage, and it could be treated.

Not again!

My world literarily just fell in front of my eyes.

I took the first plane to Houston, TX. Made an appointment with my doctor and asked him to verify the findings.

He confirmed the diagnosis. Stage 1-A Adenocarcinoma was less than an inch long.

In my first surgery in 2004, doctors removed half of my esophagus.

This time they had to take the remaining organ and tie my stomach to my larynx, making a tube that would act as an esophagus.

I was scared.

The second time around was no party. I still had difficulty with the first surgery, as my digestion had changed. But now, what could I expect?

I stopped all decisions dead. I had to breathe; I had to have a plan, and I had to do something.

I would not get this thing a third time. I would rather just give up, talk to the family about my decision, go to the seaside to live, and let nature take its course.

As I was sitting in the waiting room to see my doctor, a young man sat next to me, no more than 30. He smiled, and as I smiled back, he asked me if I was going to have surgery. I said yes, that was the plan.

"You are lucky," he said. "My cancer in the esophagus is in stage three; surgery is no longer an option."

"Why I asked,"

"Well, for one, there is metastasis. The cancer has spread through my lymphatic system, and two, they need to keep my strength up, as my treatments are very strong. I am in my third year of treatment, and I don't know how many more I will have. You have an opportunity to get well after surgery. You are lucky."

That brought me out of my self-pity.

At that moment, I decided I was going to fight.

That I would do whatever it took to not only get well but go into remission forever.

Although the tumor was small, the doctors felt they had to remove the remaining organ and try to attach the stomach, which would be reduced to a tube near my larynx.

If I had trouble with digestion, this was going to be worse.

They also recommended radiation. Chemo before the operation and after surgery.

I was in it for the long haul.

After the news, I took off some time off. I went to the seaside to reflect on my bad luck, feeling alone and lost.

I felt sorry for myself.

I felt it was unfair.

Tears kept on appearing in my eyes.

As I sat near the beach, I saw an old fisherman throwing his net, with incredible skill, and yet catching nothing. I was curious, so I stayed observing his rhythmic movements. Nothing. Just before sunset, he packed his net and started rowing toward the shore with an empty boat.

The next day, early in the morning, as the sun rose on the horizon, I saw him again, with the same movements, and the same results. He would not give up.

At one moment, I approached him and asked him if he ever caught any fish. With a big smile, he answered, "With perseverance, anything is possible."

At that point, the penny dropped. I remembered the words of the young man in the hospital "You are lucky to get an operation".

Then I decided I would not give up.

In my last surgery, I had done everything my doctors had requested.

This time, I was going to take control of my life.

I was going to take control of the outcome.

I remember I sat in the house for nearly two weeks, getting my hands on every book or article written about my cancer.

The medical journals helped little, as they were more focused on new medical treatments than on anything else.

I started reading about patients' success stories. A recurring theme formed in my mind.

It was at this point that my life changed radically.

I had to analyze my attitude toward life, my spirituality, and my environment.

It was then that I realized that after my first treatment in 2004, I went back to my old lifestyle. Nothing had changed. My life was just as chaotic as before, and cancer had just been a bump in the road.

With a new resolution in my head and my notebook, I went to face the enemy. I went into treatment with a different attitude.

This book summarizes what I did.

CHAPTER ONE

"If you know the enemy and know yourself, you need not fear the result of a hundred battles. If you know yourself but not the enemy, for every victory gained, you will also suffer a defeat. If you know neither the enemy nor yourself, you will succumb in every battle."

— **Sun Tzu, <u>The Art of War</u>**

FIRST STEP

WHAT IS CANCER?

Our body is made of approximately 60 billion cells.

These cells are constantly reproducing to take over cells that die in our organs as in blood, bones, lymphatic system, and immune system.

During the reproduction of a cell, the cell goes through a transformation called mitosis. In this process, the cell divides itself in two, making an identical copy of itself with the same genetic code. Thus, replicating itself.

Through this process, millions of cells replicate themselves constantly.

There are bound to be mistakes. Some cells that are replicated do not have the exact genetic code as the mother cell, so they become defective cells.

Normally, the immune system destroys these cells.

Unfortunately, some of these cells survive detection and continue to live in our bodies as rogue cells until either they die or they find a host where they can live. These cells can aggregate themselves in the walls or linings of the body's organs, and reproduce without control, destroying the organ.

This is the beginning of cancer.

There are over 100 types of cancer, having one thing in common; their uncontrollable reproduction and destruction of the tissues where they grow.

Cancer is named after the organs or tissue where the cells develop. Cancer can also be named after the cells they are invading and forming a tumor.

The organ usually affects the name of the cancer. Examples are **breast cancer**, prostate cancer, lung cancer, and skin cancer.

Tumors are then a swelling, or a lump produced by these cells when they reproduce abnormally.

Tumors can be benign or malignant.

Cancerous tumors can be solid or liquid.

Solid tumors normally appear in organs like the lungs, breasts, esophagus, and liver.

Liquid tumors usually form in a liquid environment, like the lymphatic system, blood, or bone marrow. These include leukemia, lymphoma, and multiple myeloma.

When we talk about cancer, certain terms are used that you should familiarize yourself with.

A **tumor,** as we have seen, can be liquid or solid, formed by cancerous cells that are reproducing uncontrollably.

When your doctor discovers a lump or mass in one of your organs, he will require a **biopsy** of the tumor, and then a pathologist will determine if it is **benign**, not cancerous, or **malignant**, or cancerous. In a biopsy, doctors remove part or the whole tumor.

Your doctor with the biopsy will determine the **grade** of the tumor, which will determine how aggressive the tumor is. The grading system goes from 1 to 4, where 1 is where the cells are very close to normal. They are defined as "**well-differentiated**". These tumor cells grow and spread slowly.

In grades 3 and 4, tumor cells do not look like normal cells surrounding the tissue. They define them as **poorly or undifferentiated**. These tumor cells proliferate and spread faster in the body.

Do not confuse the tumor grade with the **stage** of the tumor. The stages determine the size of the tumor and the possibility of it spreading to surrounding tissue. Stages go from 1 to a small tumor. Stage 4 means that it is a large tumor and that it has spread to other parts of the body.

The grading and staging systems are important because they will determine the strategy that your oncologist will follow in treating cancer. The treatment options are varied and include surgery, radiation, chemotherapy, targeted cancer drugs, hormone therapy, or a combination of them. These treatments can be accompanied by alternative therapies, also called Complementary Therapies. These relieve treatment symptoms or side effects.

It is incredibly important that if you undergo these types of complementary treatments, inform your oncologist, as you do not want them to interfere with your treatment. This has a simple explanation. If you do not inform your doctor that you are complimenting the treatment with herbs, for example, he cannot determine if the treatment drugs are doing their job or if another substance hindered them. He will then be blind to the outcome of the strategy he designed.

I used complementary supplements, and I will talk about my experience later in the book, but I assure you, my doctor knew exactly what I was taking and the doses.

The spreading of cancer cells in the body is called **metastases,** and it spreads in the body in three different ways.

First, it just simply penetrates adjoining tissue.

The second is called **hematogenous propagation,** which simply means the distribution of cancer cells through the blood system.

Third, through the lymphatic system.

This is the body's sewage system, where part of the immune cells travel with toxins and pathogens that have invaded the body. The cancer cells propagate there. They then attach themselves to the right tissue.

There are three main types of tumors, depending on where they grow.

Carcinomas. They live in the epithelial tissues of organs, specifically in the lining of organs and the body. Most of these tumors grow in tissues that secrete liquids. Milk in the breast; seminal fluid in the prostate; mucus in the lungs; gastric juices in the pancreas, and so on. This was the cancer found in the lining of my esophagus.

Sarcomas. These tumors develop in supportive or connecting tissues, like the muscles, bones, tendons, cartilage, nerves, fat, or blood vessels.

Melanomas. These are tumors arising in the pigment cells of the skin.

Lymphomas are tumors that arise from the lymphocytes, and they form in the lymphatic system, in the lymph nodes, spleen, thymus, and bone marrow. There are two types, non-Hodgkin, the most common, and Hodgkin. The difference is in the lymphocyte cells they are involved with. They do not form solid tumors.

Leukemia is a cancer of the blood. It is a cancer in the blood cells caused by a rise in the count of white cells. They crowd out the red cells and platelets your body needs to be healthy. These cancers do not form solid tumors either.

HOW IS CANCER DETECTED

The ideal time to detect cancer is in its early stages.

This is done with routine checkups. Unfortunately, we don't do it often enough.

In 2007, I went to the doctor's office to have my routine checkup. Two years had gone by, and the visits were less frequent, and I was having one every six months. I was lucky; the detection was early. I went for my checkups religiously. At the back of my mind, I had this feeling that the disease could reappear, and it did.

Unfortunately, people go to the doctor when something is not right. They visit their doctor when they feel a lump, or they are in pain.

What doctors do first is a physical exam. They feel the lymph nodes and press the area where the pain or lump has originated as in **breast cancer**. A rectal exam is necessary for the prostate, or a Papanicolaou for cervical cancer.

Your doctor will ask for a blood and urine test, for cancer or tumor markers.

Tumor markers are substances that are produced by cancer cells or other cells of the body in response to cancer or certain benign (noncancerous) situations. We can find these substances in the blood, urine, stool, tumor tissue, or other body fluids.

Your doctor and the laboratory technician will decide if these markers are high enough to do further testing, or if they deviate from the normal standards.

MEDICAL IMAGING

Medical imaging has advanced in the last five years to such a degree that it has revolutionized almost every aspect of medicine.

More detailed imaging can now allow doctors to more accurate diagnostics and determine better treatments.

Ultrasound is the safest and most cost-effective form of imaging. It uses high-frequency sound waves that are transmitted from the probe to the body via a conducting gel that bounces back at different speeds as they hit different structures within the body.

X-ray imaging. Madame Curie discovered this form of imaging in 1885. The process works with wavelengths and frequencies that penetrate the skin to create an image. Apart from using them for the visualization of skeletal tissue, it is also helpful in the diagnosis of **breast cancer** through mammography. In the digestive tissues, doctors take images with the help of barium or enemas.

Computer Tomography. Also known as CT Computer Axial Tomography or CAT scans. They are a form of X-Ray that creates a 3D image for diagnosis. The CT scanner has a large circular opening for the patient to lie on a motorized table. The X-Ray source and detector then rotate around you and create a snapshot of the body. Doctors then assembled them with the aid of computers to make one, or several, images of the internal organs. The important fact is that these images not only do they give more clarity to solid structures of the body, but they also give good imaging of soft tissue like organs, muscles, and blood vessels.

Magnetic Resonance Imaging or MRI This procedure uses magnetic fields and radio waves to generate images of the body that can penetrate inside soft tissue, as in between joints or ligaments. These procedures are usually used to examine internal body structures to diagnose strokes, tumors, spinal cord injuries, aneurysms, and brain function.

Endoscopies are nonsurgical procedures used to examine a person's internal ducts. Using an endoscope, a flexible tube with a light, and a camera attached to it, your doctor can see images of the ducts on a color tv monitor and take pictures. There are upper endoscopies that are performed for gastric duct analysis. They introduce a tube in the mouth into the esophagus, allowing your doctor to view the esophagus, stomach, and the upper part of the small intestine. Other endoscopes are introduced into the large intestine and are called colonoscopy. Doctors also use endoscopies called ERCPs (Endoscopic retrograde cholangiopancreatography) to take images of the pancreas and gallbladder.

Biopsies. During endoscopies, your surgeon might feel he has to take a sample of tissue for closer examination in a laboratory. This procedure is called a biopsy. Interventional radiologists, or interventional cardiologists, can also perform biopsies. These biopsies can take a sample of the tumor or extract the whole tumor in the intervention.

NEW TRENDS IN IMAGING

Mammography. Digital Breast Tomosynthesis (DBT) is a 3D mammography it improves lesion visibility and early cancer detection. This technology uses multiple images of the breast, enabling doctors to view each tissue layer independently, reducing the number of errors and recalls.

Ultrasonic Holography. Since ultrasonic technology does not use radiation, it is ideal for preventive and post-surgery examinations in **breast cancer** patients. The resolution of the images is significantly better than normal ultrasound, enabling doctors to review images on their computers.

WHAT CAUSES CANCER

Cancer has no one cause.

It is a combination of many factors. Cancer is not like an infection where you respond by taking a determined antibiotic. With cancer, it's not that easy. Studies of the disease have confirmed that the most common factors are:

Toxic Overload.

As governments and Agro-industry are pressured by the growth of population, and the cultivation areas reduced, they have resorted to chemicals in plants to conserve and increase yield.

Unfortunately, pests mutate just as fast as we develop new pesticides and worst, pests become immune to many of the chemicals that are used. Only in the US, there are approximately 80 thousand chemicals registered. We are directly in contact with over 60 thousand, of which 20 thousand are carcinogens. The government has banned many of these chemicals, yet other countries still permit them.

Will we import products from these countries?

We already do. Especially from Asia.

A study done in Canada by the College of Family Physicians of Canada showed a "positive association between cancer and pesticides" as reported in The National Library of Medicine[i]

These chemicals then accumulate in our bodies, not only affecting the DNA of our cells but also affecting our immune system and increasing chronic inflammation in our body. With a weak immune system, cancer cells run free in our bodies.

Stress Although researchers have not proven that stress is a direct cause of cancer, the community widely accepts that stress affects tumor growth and metastasis in cancer patients.

The National Cancer Institute published this, in an article "Psychological Stress and Cancer" as reported by the National Cancer Institute[ii] stating that there is evidence from experimental studies to suggest that psychological stress can affect a tumor's ability to grow and spread.

In 1936, Dr. Hans Style showed in Canada that there was a correlation between stressed rats and the shrinkage of the thymus gland. This experiment was then corroborated in February 2005 and published in Science Direct. [iii]

The thymus gland is a gland in our throats that, apart from the production of certain hormones, also plays a crucial role in the production of "T" cells for the immune system. The shrinkage of the gland seriously compromises the production of these cells, affecting our entire immune system, and letting cancer cells run rampant in our bodies.

Nutrition. Our body is made, repaired, and fed by substances that are found in the diet. Regrettably, our modern style of life, "eating on the run," has given us less time to eat a home-cooked meal and more processed food. It is much easier to cook in the microwave than to prepare the entire meal from zero. Unfortunately, most of these quick meals are lacking basic nutritional ingredients and more added substances to make them keep longer and taste better. The constant consumption of these processed products has created a nutritional deficient generation. It has also created a generation that is more prone to chronic diseases, like diabetes, cancer, asthma, arthritis, cystic fibrosis, and others.

Sedentary Lifestyle. The numbers are overwhelming. The National Cancer Institute published "Cancer Statistics" in 2020, stating that over 1.8 million cancer cases were expected in 2020. Of these, 70% were expected to survive for five or more years as reported by the American Cancer Society. [iv] They also published an article in May 2016 linking exercise and the lower incidence of 13 types of cancer. They recommended 150 minutes of moderate-intensity or 75 vigorous walking each week. This was great news, as we had an excellent incentive to become active again. [v]

Researchers widely understand the relationship between cancer and exercise. Exercise helps circulation and the distribution of oxygen to the cells. Blood also distributes white cells, for a better defense against pathogens and cancer cells. Exercise stabilizes the levels of glucose in the blood, which helps to "starve" cancerous cells.

Cancer and Genetics. Many of us know somebody that has had cancer. Some are family members. Yet, more than half of the cancers that appear are sporadic. It means they appear influenced by other factors, not by genetics.

Sporadic Cancer. Is a cancer that appears for reasons other than genetics.

Familial Cancer. These are cancers caused by a combination of genetics and environmental risk factors.

Hereditary cancers. These appear when an altered gene is passed down in the family. Mutations in DNA that are harmful may increase a person's chance or risk of developing cancer. Overall, inherited mutations play a role in about 5% of all cancers.

It is difficult to pinpoint the direct causes of cancer, yet it is important to understand that if you inherit a modified gene, it does not mean that you are doomed to get cancer; it means that the RISK has increased by 50% approximately, and if you have a healthy lifestyle, it is highly improbable that you will get cancer. Genetic testing has become more relevant, as reported in the National Library of Medicine. Talk to your doctor if you need more information. [vi]

The Immune system. We all have cancer cells in our bodies. Yes, it is a frightening idea, yet it is a fact. Not all cancer cells grow to be tumors. Our immune system takes care of that.

Organs compose our bodies, functioning independently. They keep the harmony of functions as if they were working together, keeping us healthy. The most incredible system in the body is the immune system. It is comparable to the body's laws and orders together with the army. These cells' sole function is to control and destroy, when necessary, the invasions of external pathogens and mutated cells in the body. They are constantly cleaning our bodies of bacteria, viruses, and other invaders like fungi and parasites.

The first line of defense of the immune system is the mucous membranes, the skin, and the stomach acid. All these create a defense system that stops external pathogens from entering the body.

The second line of defense includes the inflammatory response and the phagocytes. These appear when bacteria, injured tissues, trauma, toxins, heat, or other causes affect our bodies. The damaged cells release immediately chemicals that include histamine, bradykinin, and prostaglandins. These chemicals cause blood vessels to leak fluid into the damaged tissue, causing swelling. This process isolates the area from the rest of the adjoining tissue, preventing further damage. The chemicals also attract white blood cells called "phagocytes" that engulf and "eat" germs and dead or damaged cells. Phagocytes eventually die, forming pus with other dead cells.

SUMMARY

What is cancer?

- Cancer is many afflictions of the cellular system, and not just one.
- The common factor is that these afflictions affect the cells to reproduce uncontrollably.
- These cells survive the immune system and can act as normal cells.
- The cancer is named after the organ it affects. Breast, lung, prostate, and others.

Tumor. Is an abnormal mass of tissue that can be solid or fluid filled.

Benign Tumor. A non-cancerous tumor.

Malignant Tumor. A cancerous tumor.

Biopsy. A sample of tissue is taken from the body in order

to analyze it.

Metastasis. Cells break from the primary source and travel in the bloodstream or lymphatic system to other parts of the body.

Tumor Grade. From 1 to 4, shows how aggressive is the growth of the tumor.

Cancer stage. Is a measure to determine how much cancer is in the body, tumor size, and where it is located. It also describes the extent the cancer has spread in the body.

Types of cancer.

- Carcinomas. Cancer that grows in the lining of organs or skin.
- Sarcoma. Cancer that grows in connecting tissue.
- Lymphoma. Cancer that grows in the lymphoid tissue. Two main types are Hodgkin and non-Hodgkin.
- Leukemia. Cancer that grows in the blood system.

Cancer diagnosis.

- Physical exam.
- Blood Tests, to determine markers.

Imaging

- Ultrasound. AZ method uses high-frequency sound waves.
- X-ray. Imaging through high-frequency electromagnetic radiation.
- Pet Scan. Positron Emission Tomography.
- MIR. Magnetic Resonance Imaging, using magnetic fields.

Endoscopy.

The use of a flexible tube with a camera is introduced in the body's cavities, usually in the esophagus, stomach, small intestine, and colon.

What causes cancer?

Not just one thing. Cancer is a sum of various afflictions that cause cells to mutate and grow uncontrollably in the body. Factors that influence the mutation of cells are toxic overdose, stress, nutrition, sedentary lifestyle, and genetic factors.

CHAPTER TWO

"Attack is the secret of defense;
defense is the planning of an attack."
— **Sun Tzu, <u>The Art of War</u>**

SECOND STEP

PLANNING

People are shocked when they are told they have cancer. With reason. Everybody would be, even if you are a medical professional. Nothing prepares you for that piece of news. This is called trauma. You will go through various phases of trauma, namely shock, denial, anger, and acceptance. It is a process, so let it happen. Go through the phases and live them. This is how we will process the news. We want these phases to pass by swiftly. In my case, it took around a week. Although my adenocarcinoma developed quickly, the doctors said I could take some time off.

With shock comes fear, which dulls your mind. You do not know what to do. Then comes negation and denial. "The doctor is wrong" and "This cannot happen to me". These affirmations are good if you take action. Get a second opinion. Funnily this action will make you feel better. Because now you are being proactive. If the doctors confirm your diagnosis, then there will be anger. Anger with life, God, yourself, etc. This is normal. The mind does not like that you have left your comfort zone.

Then acceptance will appear. This is the tipping point. There are two types of acceptance. Passive acceptance, where you become an object of medical procedure, and you do exactly what you are told, waiting for the moment this nightmare ends. Then you go back to your old way of life. The other is active acceptance, where you take control of your life. You let doctors do what they are experts at, yet you talk to them about your body, not a statistic and a protocol, your BODY, and how it reacts and feels. You are the expert there.

Take your time in this process, but not too long, as you will have to sit down with your team to plan a strategy.

Build a team. The first thing to do is to choose a doctor you trust and the way he explains things to you. That he has the patience to let you explore options and listen to you. He will be your Medical Coordinator. He doesn't have to be your oncologist or your surgeon, or even your radiologist, although it helps if he has a specialty in these fields.

You will then ask him to be your medical team leader, meaning that he can coordinate most of the medical procedures and explain them to you. He will become your best friend. You will still need to see your oncologist or radiologist, but they will coordinate with your doctor, and he will help you decide the best way to go. Don't forget to advise your surgeon, oncologist, or radiologist that your doctor is coordinating your procedures. This will let them know you are being guided by your primary physician, and that they can discuss the treatments in their language.

It is important to name a medical team leader, because then you can deposit all your medical decisions and treatment strategies on him, and you can concentrate your effort on getting well and taking control of your life.

Family and friends. Find an associate for this journey. It is ideal if it is your spouse or a close family member. Beware, sometimes these can become bossy and start telling you what to do. Remember, the objective is to take control of your life. Select a partner, somebody who listens, who will be there when you are down, who will encourage you on your journey, who will help you mentally and physically. This person will help you coordinate friends and family chores. They will take you to your treatments, will help you with prescriptions, and take care of insurance and finances. In the beginning, you will feel quite independent, yet as the treatments advance, you will feel tired, and you will appreciate somebody taking care of tedious things.

This family leader will also handle all queries from family members and friends. There is nothing more annoying and depressing than having to tell the same story repeatedly or listening to somebody else's experience. Block all that out. You are different and your body is unique.

Once you have your family team, get them all together and inform them of the plan. Make them part of your strategy and let them commit to your well-being.

Your family leader will meet with all your friends and inform them of the situation and what is the strategy. During these reunions, you will get a lot of offers of help, and your leader should try to organize them. Don't do it yourself. You will be just burdening your mind with details that somebody else will take care of.

Your Family leader will then open a notebook, where she/he will keep tabs on medicines, medical exams, imaging, timetables, exercise routines, meals, physical and mental status, who does what, and when. A journal of your illness. This will be extremely helpful when talking to doctors about the reactions to the treatment and your progress.

Questions to keep in mind when visiting your oncologist.

- How accurate is the diagnostic testing?
- Can you help me get a second opinion?
- Where is my cancer and has it spread?
- Will I need surgery, and what can I expect?
- What kind of treatment do you suggest and what results can we expect?
- What is the treatment aiming to achieve?
- What could be the potential side effects?

- Will you have a plan to treat side effects, including pain?
- How will you know if the treatment is working?
- Do you recommend special nutrition?
- How long will these treatments go for?
- When will it be important to call your office?
- Where will the treatments, appointments, and tests be?
- Do you believe in alternative treatments?
- Can I take supplements?
- How will you maintain my immune system at its optimum?
- Are there any clinical trials I should look at?
- Will I need chemotherapy?
- What drugs will I be receiving and how will they be administered?
- How many treatments, and for how long?
- How strong will the side effects be?
- Is there anything I can do to lessen the effects?
- What do I do if I have severe side effects? Who do I call?
- Will I be able to go to work during the whole treatment?
- Does my insurance cover the cost of treatment?
- Will I benefit from support groups? Which do you recommend?
- How will the success of the treatment be assessed and how?

When you visit your oncologist, be sure your family leader goes with you and takes notes on all answers.

You might have additional questions. Do not keep them to yourself, even if you feel they are trivial.

What's important is to feel comfortable with the answers and you are confident of the outcome.

Questions you should ask your surgeon.

- What procedure will you use?
- Are there any alternatives?
- What potential dangers are there?
- What kind of anesthetic is going to be used?
- Are there any risks associated with anesthesia?
- Will it be an open procedure or a minimally invasive one?
- What medications will be administered before the procedure?
- When should I stop eating before the procedure?
- Is there anything I should do to speed recovery?
- Will I need to arrange for help while recovering?
- Will I be able to drive home?
- How will the pain be managed?
- How long will I be in the hospital?
- When will I be able to exercise?
- When will I be able to eat and drink after surgery?

Questions you should ask your radiologist.

- How does radiation work?

- What type of radiation will I receive?
- Will you make permanent or temporary set-up marks?
- Where will I receive treatment?
- How long will the sessions take?
- How many treatments will I need?
- What are the side effects?
- How can I best handle side effects?
- How flexible is the radiation schedule?
- Can I work while receiving radiation?
- Are there any restrictions during treatment?
- If my side effects are severe, who do I call?

SUMMARY

Preparation. After getting diagnosed, you will transit through phases of trauma. Shock, Denial, Anger, and then Acceptance. Get through these as fast as possible and take control of all your actions and decisions. Ask for a second opinion. This will help you be proactive.

Build a team. Choose a medical leader. A family and friends' leader. They will be an important part of your journey.

Question your oncologist. Ask your oncologist all pertinent questions regarding your tumor, treatments, effects of treatments, alternative treatments, nutrition, and outcome.

CHAPTER THREE

"Every battle is won before it's ever fought."
— Sun Tzu, The Art of War

THIRD STEP

PREPARATION

Once you've dealt with all decisions for treatment and you have decided on a strategy with your medical leader, you will need to prepare your body and mind.

Mental Attitude or Mindset. This is the most important part of your preparation.

It's the way you will look at your illness. It's how you will combat the onslaught. Courage comes from adversity. You will get the strength to face the next session and the next depression. You will become a warrior and win all the time.

Of all the successful patients I have interviewed, this was a common factor. **Mental Attitude**. It is a complex action, yet it is simple to implement. The best way I can explain it is just by asking yourself these questions: What do I think about my future? Will I take all this laying down? Or will I fight this with all my strength? Is this illness going to win? Or am I going to win?

The power is in your decision.

The power is in your attitude.

The power is in your mind.

Each decision that you will make will give you control. To control your life step by step.

Yet you must decide. Commit yourself.

Look at the mirror, and say, "I´m going to beat this thing!" "I´m going to win!"

Once you decide, all your doubts and anxieties will fade away.

They will sometimes appear throughout the treatment, but you will be committed to winning.

Share with your team your commitment, because not only will they join you in the commitment, but it will give them the strength to face cancer with you.

If you don't do this for yourself, then do it for your loved ones. They are also suffering, as they do not know how to react. They want to help, and to keep loving you. The best gift you can give them is a simple message: I am going to fight this.

Prepare your body for the fight. The principal aim is to prepare your body and your mind for the physical trauma they will go through. Chemotherapy, radiation, and surgery are controlled traumas that the body will undergo. These treatments aim to destroy cancer cells as fast as possible. Unfortunately, these treatments are not very selective, and they also destroy healthy cells. Chemotherapy is introduced in the body, and it affects all areas. Radiation, although more directed, also affects adjoining tissues. Surgery is the most invasive, affecting the immune system in such a way that it depletes our defenses.

To counter all these effects, prepare your body.

You will need to make some minor changes in your lifestyle a few weeks before and during the treatments.

Forget about alcohol and tobacco. These two products are poison to your system and will seriously affect the homeostasis of your body: its balance.

Alcohol turns into sugars in the body and sugars feed cancer.

Don't consume refined sugars. This is one enemy to fight. Just analyze this. When doctors do an MRI to find out where your cancer is located, they inject a radioactive glucose solution. Why do you think this is? Glucose feeds cancer cells, and most of the solution will concentrate around your tumor, where the MRI will pick it up. Believe me, it is crucial. Give up refined sugars. I will talk a bit more about this subject later in the book.

Drink water. Get in the habit of doing this. It is incredible how often this important fact is overlooked. It is well known to doctors that many of their patients arrive for treatment completely dehydrated and they do not know it. Water is essential to our bodies. So, always keep a glass of water next to you. Take a bottle of water wherever you go. Your body will thank you during your treatment. Please avoid sodas, canned juice, fruits, and sports drinks. These have sugar added to them, especially the sports drinks that have added glucose. As we have seen, sugar feeds cancer.

Drink green tea. Exchange your coffee for green tea. This Asian beverage is a cancer patient's best friend. It has antioxidants that help eliminate free radicals. It has phytochemicals that help to stop the spreading of cancer cells, and the formation of blood vessels to feed tumors.

Fruits and veggies. Increase your consumption of these in your daily meals and reduce red meats.

Get out of the couch. Get in the habit of walking at a brisk pace 20 minutes a day. At one point, it will be difficult, yet it is important. Do it during treatment, as it helps the circulatory system get the medication around the whole body. Exercise produces endorphins which help you mentally, reducing anxiety and depression.

SUMMARY

Mental attitude. This is one of the most important action items. Your mental attitude will determine how you will face this illness. Will you just give up and let destiny take its course? Or will you commit to fighting this illness, to end it? This is your choice. This is your prerogative. I promise you, if you decide to become a warrior, you will feel better and see the light at the end of the tunnel.

Before treatment. Prepare yourself mentally and physically. Your mind and your body will have to be in optimum shape. Your body will have to face the onslaught of chemotherapy, radiation, and surgery. You need to be in top shape.

Avoid. Tobacco, alcohol, and sugar. These are our society's legal poisons. Keep away from them, they only help cancer cells to prosper.

Add water to your diet. Water, pure water, no soft drinks, sugary canned juices, and sports drinks. They all contain sugar that feeds cancer cells. Exchange coffee for green tea, its ingredients help to kill cancer cells. Add more veggies and fruits to your diet. Their phytochemical structure will help the body boost the immune system and provide essential vitamins and minerals for the optimum function of the body's organs.

Exercise. Get out of the couch. Move. Get your blood flowing and breathe deep. You will feel better. You only need 20 minutes of brisk walking a day. How hard can that be?

CHAPTER FOUR

"Your positive future begins at this moment. All you have is right now. Every goal is possible from here."

— **Lao Tsu**

FOURTH STEP

TREATMENTS

Conventional treatments.

Surgery, radiation, chemotherapy, hormonal therapy, and biological therapy. These are the primary treatments that are used universally. Surgery and radiation are treatments that focus on the tumor and its position. While chemotherapy, hormonal and biological therapies are systemic, meaning that they are administered so that they travel through the blood system to the whole body. For most cancers, a combination of these treatments is used.

Your oncologist will be the doctor that will determine what strategy to follow. Sometimes surgery, then chemo and radiation. Sometimes chemo and radiation before surgery. It all depends on the type of cancer, stage, and grade. The goal of these treatments is to cure the illness and to control the growth of the tumor, or to mitigate the pain. It is dependent on your particular situation. Your oncologist and your medical leader will discuss the strategy.

TIP

Keep a journal. Write down medicines, timetables, treatments, nutrition and how you are feeling. This will help your doctor in your meetings.

Radiation therapy.

This procedure treats the tumor with high-energy waves or particles. Radiologists focus them on the tumor, and as they pass through the body, they destroy not only the cancer cells but also collaterally healthy cells. Yet healthy cells can replace damaged tissue faster and go back to their original functions. The doctors carefully program radiation to focus on its target and minimize collateral damage.

Commonly, radiation is administered by an external beam and focused through a linear accelerator, delivering high-energy x-rays or electrons to the region of the tumor.

Before the treatment, a simulation session will be required to program the process. You will lie on a table and with the aid of a computerized tomography (CT) your oncology radiologist will determine where the tumor is and its surrounding organs, mapping the tumor and adjacent tissue. This will give them enough information to plan your treatment. To keep you still and at the right angle of beam delivery, some cushions might be used. They will mark the beam area with a small tattoo the size of a pin.

Once they determine your strategy, they will program your sessions five days a week for 1 to 10 weeks. The amount of treatments depends on the type of cancer.

Each session takes about 10 to 30 minutes. It is painless. During the weekend, you will have no therapy and it will give time for your normal cells to restore.

During a session, you will communicate with the radiation team through an intercom.

When the cycle concludes, your oncologist will require further imaging to see the progress of the radiation. This will give them an insight into the efficacy of the treatment by analyzing what changes to make.

For any discomfort arising from the treatment, discuss it with your doctor, even if the discomfort is menial.

An internal device can also administer radiation. This is called **Brachytherapy** where a radiation source such as a seed, ribbon, or tube is inserted inside the body of the tumor, or close to it. They can leave the source inside the body from minutes to days.

Other forms of radiation can be when taken orally or injected in the vein. Sometimes in these procedures, you will need to stay in the hospital for observation.

Chemotherapy.

This treatment involves chemical substances to destroy cancer cells.

Unfortunately, it also damages healthy cells. Especially in the fast-growing tissues, such as the lining of the mouth, bone marrow, gastrointestinal duct, hair, etc.

Therefore, there are several side effects to this treatment that we shall address later.

Cancer cells with this treatment simply die. Healthy cells also die, but they grow back, and tissues become normal.

The side effects of chemicals are less severe than they were 15 years ago.

There are over 100 types of cancers detected in the last few years. Your oncologist will analyze you to determine what type of cancer you are suffering from and prescribe the correct chemicals to be used.

If you receive chemo before surgery, the aim will be to reduce as much as possible the tumor, to extract it completely without fear of spilling cells in the surrounding tissue.

Doctors must leave no cancer cells behind after surgery, so they might prescribe chemo after surgery.

Sometimes, they prescribe chemo before and after surgery.

The intravenous infusion usually administers chemo. Doctors give you the drug by inserting a tube with a needle into the vein in your hand, or arm, or into a device in a vein in your chest.

When doctors use an injection in the vein, the process can take only a minute. They can also give it in a form of a drip. This process can last hours.

Nowadays more and more doctors are prescribing oral chemo. They can be in a liquid or capsule. When administering this way, you will have to be very strict with the timetables and doses, the reason being that the drugs must maintain a certain level of presence in the body to be effective.

The chemo cycles can be daily, weekly, or monthly. After the cycle, you will rest. They can repeat the cycles up to 6 times. Sometimes they will go on for an entire year.

Periodically, your oncologist will want to see the progress, so he will request imaging. CTs or MRIs and others. You will need blood tests to maintain an eye on blood cell counts and to ensure that your immune system does not become too weak to fight off infections.

Vascular Access Devices (VAD) Doctors insert them into veins via peripheral or central vessels for the administration of drugs during an extended period. To save the patient from constant piercing, these are used to access the bloodstream.

These can be catheters or ports.

Catheters are long, narrow hollow tubes made of soft plastic that are inserted every three days or weekly.

Ports or port-a-cath, is a disc the size of a quarter that is placed under your skin. They connect this device to a large vein in your chest or upper arm, to distribute the drugs faster.

Catheters and ports have special care, so ask your medical team what to do.

In my case, doctors inserted a subcutaneous port in my chest connected to the right internal jugular vein. This was more comfortable, as I am a little apprehensive about needles. The port was used to draw blood and administer chemo in the hospital. Also, when I had to carry a small infuser bottle for long periods while I was at home.

Hormonal Therapy.

The hormones are substances produced by glands that are transported to distant organs to regulate their functions and behavior.

Some hormones encourage the growth of some cancers, such as certain types of **breast cancer** and prostate cancer. Hormone therapy usually involves the taking of certain drugs that prevent or slow the production of hormones that stimulate cancer growth.

The hormone testosterone, which is produced primarily by the testis, is the primary cause of this cancer and stimulates prostate cancer. The therapy aims to stop the production of testosterone.

In some extreme cases, they remove the testicles (orchiectomy). The side effects of this procedure can include small breast growth, low sexual desire, erectile dysfunction, weight gain, and fatigue.

Sometimes estrogen, a female hormone produced in the ovaries, stimulated cancer cells in the breast. In this case, hormone therapy uses medicines that affect breast-cancer cells by lowering the amount of estrogen in the body, or by blocking the stimulation of estrogen on cancer cells.

It is important to notice that hormone therapy is not effective if the cancer cells are hormone receptor negative, meaning that hormones do not stimulate them.

There are several types of medicines used, including selective estrogen-receptors modulators: estrogen-receptors down regulators, and aromatase inhibitors. Aromatase is an enzyme that is fundamental in the production of estrogen. Inhibiting this enzyme ensures the reduction of estrogen in the body. Sometimes, the ovaries and fallopian tubes may be surgically removed. The ovaries can be also temporarily closed down with medicines. Some of the side effects are hot flashes, irritation, vaginal secretion, and fatigue.

Biological therapy.

Also called biotherapy or immunotherapy, and these include several ways to treat cancer by stimulating the immune system. Some treatments are:

Monoclonal antibodies. These recognize a specific abnormal protein that attaches itself to the surface of the cancerous cell, identifying them and attacking them directly. Chemo or radioactive isotopes may accompany this treatment.

Cytokines. These are small proteins that destroy cancerous cells or stimulate the immune system. Interferon is an example of this. Animal cells produce these specific proteins in response to the entry of a virus. These proteins have the property of inhibiting the reproduction of cancer cells. One other property is that it stimulates killer "T" cells in the immune system, to attack cancer cells.

Vaccines. They produce them with changed and inactive cancer cells that, when introduced into the patient's body, activate the immune system to produce antibodies to destroy that specific cancer cell.

Recent laboratory studies as published in Nature Cancer Papers on 10th November 2022, led by researchers Lei Tiang and Bo Xu, have found that activating tumors with oncolytic viruses makes the tumors more vulnerable to immunotherapy as published. Nature Cancer Papers 10 November 2022.[vii]

Surgery

Surgery serves various purposes:

- To diagnose. Surgeons take a small sample to determine if the tissue is cancerous. It also determines the type of cancer and the rate of growth or stage. This procedure is called a biopsy. Sometimes during a biopsy, they examine the area around the tumor, including the lymph nodes, to determine how far cancer has spread and to establish its "stage".

- Primary Surgery. This is done when they find the cancer in a specific part of the body. Its accessibility permits the removal of the entire tumor. Here, chemo or radiation can accompany the surgery.

- Debulking surgery is done when not all the tumor can be removed because of its position or invasion of important organs. Surgeons remove the main body of the tumor, and they attack the remaining part with chemo and radiation.

- Palliative surgery is done for patients with advanced cancer. Its main purpose is to ease pain and discomfort caused by the tumor, by eliminating the causing factors, yet they do not attack the tumor itself.

- Reconstructive surgery is used to improve a person's looks after major cancer surgery. It is also used to restore the functions of organs that were affected. Breast reconstruction is an example of this procedure.

- Prophylactic surgery. Surgeons take this option to remove body tissue that is likely to become cancerous. The tissue may not have any signs of cancer, but it is likely to be invaded.

Most cancers, if not all, will need a biopsy to diagnose them. Doctors only performed major cancer surgery in 67% of the cases.

NEW CONVENTIONAL TREATMENTS.

Traditionally, the most common form of treatment for cancer in our times is chemotherapy, radiotherapy, tumor surgery, and with breast and prostate cancer, hormonal therapy.

However, other types of treatments are surfacing in combination with traditional treatments. The aim is to eradicate cancer cells from the body as fast as possible and with fewer side effects.

The most recent cancer research breakthroughs are:

Immunotherapy. The aim is to boost the immune system for it to combat cancer cells. The problem is that some cancer cells pass undetected by the immune system, and they thrive with no hindrance. Other cancer cells go further and promote the immune system by helping them develop.

In an article in Nature Immunology published in 2017, scientists found that some white cells failed to identify cancer cells because these produced two signals to the white cells meant to repel their destroying action. These reactions showed scientists the way to creating ways to block the signals created by the cancer cells, thus the white cells, or macrophages, can identify the cancer cells and destroy them.

In Great Britain, a team of scientists is using a surprising alternative approach: viruses. A benign virus called reovirus is used to attack brain cancer cells while leaving healthy cells alone.

Another form of immunotherapy is the "Dendritic Vaccines". What scientists do is they collect dendritic cells from the immune system of a person, arm these cells with specific antigens, or toxins, and then they inject them back into the patient's body, to attack cancer cells.

Scientists have proven these treatments to work best when used together with chemotherapy.

Nanotechnology. Another form of treatment is using nanoparticles. These are microscopic particles that are used to target tumors while leaving healthy tissue alone. They load these particles with chemicals that destroy cancer cells. In Great Britain and China, scientists have loaded particles with substances that could expose tumors to heat while avoiding healthy tissue.

In another study, nanoprobes were used to identify micrometastases, or secondary tumors that are so small that you cannot detect them any other way.

Immunotherapy is a promising area of treatment, and what is important is that it uses your system to help destroy cancer.

Tumor Starvations. Researchers have discovered two substances that feed cancer: Glutamine, and vitamin B2. By blocking cancer cells with these two nutrients, researchers could increase the impact of oxidative stress, which kills cancer cells.

Epigenetics. This is the study of changes in organisms caused by a modification of gene expression rather than the alteration of the genetic code itself. Epigenetic factors cause many cancers and their behavior. This has given researchers a path to follow.

Targeted Cancer treatment. Of all the new cancer treatments, Target Cancer treatment is the most advanced. These treatments are drugs that block the growth and spreading, interfering with specific molecules in cancer activity.

The Food and Drug Administration (FDA) has approved many targeted therapies and they include:

- **Hormonal therapies**. These slow or stop the growth of hormonal-sensitive tumors that require these hormones to grow. They use mainly treatments for prostate and **breast cancer**.
- **Signal transduction inhibitors**. These therapies block the activity of molecules that take part in the signaling between cells and their environment. What these therapies do is interfere with the signaling between cancer cells that are reproducing uncontrollably.
- **Apoptosis inducers.** These chemicals induce the cancer cell to commit apoptosis or death.
- **Gene expression modulators**. These, as we have seen, are treatments that change the way certain genes behave, inducing cancer.
- **Angiogenesis inhibitors.** All tumors, when they get to a specific size, they need vessels to deliver nutrients for their growth. The inhibitors block the substances

that stimulate the growth of vessels to the tumor, thus killing the cells of starvation.

With new treatments, you must discuss with your oncologist and your medical leader ALL the possibilities, so you know that whatever you decide as the strategy to combat this illness is the best for you, and you alone.

CLINICAL TRIALS.

Clinical trials are research studies done on people. An institution conducts these to find alternative forms of improving treatments and quality of life for the patient.

The studies concentrate on testing new ways to treat cancer, find, and diagnose cancer, prevent cancer, and manage symptoms, and side effects of treatments.

The trials are the last step in years of analysis of drugs proven successful in the laboratory. Clinical trials are for every stage of cancer, and not only for advanced cases. The best way to find a clinical trial designed for you is to consult your health provider or visit www.cancer.gov and look for "Find NCI-Supported Clinical Trials".

Clinical trials are important for doctors to determine whether new treatments are safe and effective. When you take part, you add to the knowledge about cancer, and you help yourself in finding new ways to fight your disease.

In my case, I took part in a clinical trial where they gave me a drug to mitigate the harm radiation does to neighboring organs. As my cancer was in the esophagus, my heart and lungs were at risk. I didn't know if I was taking the drug or a placebo. But in the end, my lungs and heart were healthy, after ten weeks of radiation.

SIDE EFFECTS OF CHEMOTHERAPY AND RADIATION

Unfortunately, chemotherapy not only attacks cancer cells. It also attacks healthy cells, especially those cells with rapid reproductions. The effects depend on the drugs administered and the duration of the treatment. These side effects normally occur temporarily, and the tissues restore themselves in time.

The most common side effects are:

Hair Loss. With some chemicals, this is inevitable. The drugs attack the hair follicles, and they stop reproducing, causing hair loss. It is important to ask your oncologist if the drug that he prescribes will cause this side effect, to prepare yourself. Hair loss will occur from the 7th day to the 21st. Yet it will start growing back at the end of the treatment. Meanwhile, there are some things you can do.

- Consider cutting your hair very short, to accustom yourself to this new look. At one point, when hair loss starts, you might shave all your head and wear scarves or wigs. Some men keep their look after treatment.
- Use mild shampoos and soft brushes.

- Do not use hair blowers, especially with hot air.
- Protect your scalp from the sun. Use hats or scarves.
- Do not despair. This is a badge of honor for the treatment. Use it proudly. You are battling this disease and you will win.

When I finished my treatments, the second time around, my hair which used to be dark brown grew white and straight, not that yours will. People who knew me and hadn't seen me for a long time used to comment on my new look. When asked how I had achieved it, my answer invariably was chemotherapy. A sour joke. This had many effects. Some laughed, yet most saw that I got through the ordeal as a winner. That made me, my family, and my friends feel good. Mission accomplished.

Fatigue. This is the most common side effect. The drugs used in chemotherapy and radiation caused this. Also, by an aggressive surgery, lack of sleep, or emotional stress. Pre-existing diseases, like diabetes, thyroid problems, high blood pressure, and rheumatoid arthritis, to name a few, can also cause it.

There are certain things you can do to counter this effect.

- Exercise regularly. This is tough. When fatigue hits you, going for a walk is the last thing you want to do. But believe me, even if you feel your legs can't hold you up, do it. Get somebody to accompany you and hold you if necessary. The benefits of this will help you with the treatments. You will sleep better, the drugs will distribute themselves throughout your body, and mentally it will help you with depression, as you will concentrate on the exercise and not on how you feel.

- Limit your naps to only 30 minutes a day. Too much nap time will affect your nighttime.
- Do not drink alcohol and caffeine. No nicotine, and no chocolate. I am sorry.
- Turn the TV one hour before bedtime.
- Maintain a routine every day, in waking, eating, napping, and working. Do this on weekends too.
- Keep a diary beside your bed, and anything that is bothering you, write it down and leave it till tomorrow.
- If the fatigue is extreme. Your doctor will know what to do. In my case, the doctors took me off radiation before I finished the cycle. Yes, this was nearly 14 years ago. Now, the treatments are not as debilitating as they used to be.

Nausea. This is another common effect. It does not affect everybody, and its intensity varies. Nausea is something that you must control. Do not endure it without your doctor knowing, because nausea has two important effects.

You will stop eating properly. You will start skipping meals. This will affect your diet and reduce the nutrients that your body needs. Do not use this as an excuse to lose weight. This is not the time to do it. Your body needs every inch of help to survive the attack by these treatments.

You will also skip drinking liquids. If nausea is severe, you will probably feel like vomiting and dehydration is a big possibility. Drinking liquids, preferably water, is highly recommended, as liquids will help your body rid itself of all drugs and toxins the treatment brings with them. Check the color of your urine. You are dehydrated if the color of your urine is yellow or brownish.

Luckily, I did not have severe nausea, although I drank *ginger tea* every day. That helped a lot. Do not take supplements unless your doctor allows them. It is difficult for doctors to monitor your treatment with drugs, and it will confuse them if you add supplements to your diet. In my case, my doctor was ok with me taking supplements, so I drank *ginger tea*, whenever I felt nausea coming.

Pain. This is one of the most debilitating effects of cancer. With technology and medical advances, doctors can manage it. Pain not only affects the body, but it also affects the psyche and your state of mind. If you do not address pain, it will affect the way you view your illness and the amount of energy you will have to fight it. When I was to undergo treatment, my medical coordinator advised me to seek an algologist (pain doctor), so I did. This was probably the best decision I made as I went through surgery, radiation, and chemotherapy painlessly. I remember seeing similar patients whose doctor had not recommended this specialist, and who were struggling with their pain, especially after surgery.

Cancer by itself, not always causes pain. Sometimes it appears as a dull feeling in parts of your body, and this is when some tumors are pressing against principal organs. Yet pain also helps to diagnose cancer. When you feel it in your body and is bothersome, you normally visit your doctor. That's when doctors diagnose cancer.

Some people will feel that taking medication for pain is a sign of weakness, some others feel that if they take medications for pain, it will interfere with medication taken for cancer treatment. Nothing can be further from the truth. Your doctor will consult your oncologist or surgeon, and together they will decide what is the best way to stop you from suffering. Do not think that you deserve this illness and that dealing with pain is a punishment. Cancer is not a punishment; it is an illness that needs to be eradicated from your body. That's all. Another myth is people should take painkillers only as a last resort. They feel that if they take the medicine when the pain appears, it won't work when it gets worse. This is untrue. If you talk to an algologist, he will explain that pain should be mitigated before it appears. This way, the nervous pathway of pain that goes into our central nervous system is blocked, and the patient will feel no pain.

Pruritus. Itchy skin. This can appear in one spot, or it can cover a larger portion of the body. This effect appears for various reasons. The most common is radiation. Some of the chemo drugs can cause itching in the whole body, because of an allergic reaction. It is important to talk to your oncologist, radiologist, or health provider about this reaction, as they will have to analyze the cause and treat it accordingly. If it is an allergic reaction, the doctor will probably change the drug that is causing it. If it is radiation, the doctor will prescribe a topical cream to relieve the itching on the skin. Do not scratch. Remember that your immune system is compromised, and an infection can easily appear. Some recommendation is to bathe in lukewarm water and use neutral soaps, with no perfume. Keep your skin hydrated with creams recommended by your health provider and drink plenty of liquids.

Mouth Sores. Mucous cells are fast-growing cells, in the mouth's lining and the esophagus, for example, hence they are the first to be affected by chemotherapy. Mucositis or mouth sores appear in the mouth's lining, lips, and sometimes gums. Radiation can also cause damage, and this makes it difficult for your mouth to heal itself. It can also impair the immune system so that viruses and bacteria can more easily infect your mouth, causing mouth sores or making them worse. Bone marrow transplants and targeted therapies can also cause mouth sores.

When planning your treatments, ask your doctor if the drugs he will use cause mouth sores, and whether you should try preventive measures. Your doctor might ask you to do the following:

Get a dental checkup. Visiting your dentist before you begin cancer treatment is one of the best things you can do. Any dental issue such as cavities or gum disease will only get worse during treatment.

Tell your doctor if you have a history of mouth sores. If you have had recurring mouth sores because of the herpes simplex virus, advise him, as he can prescribe some antiviral medication.

Do not drink alcohol or smoke.

Eat plenty of fruit and vegetables. Their nutrients will help you fight off infection.

Your doctor might prescribe a coating agent which coats the whole lining of the mouth, forming a protective film around the sores and preventing further damage.

They can also prescribe some topical painkillers.

If there is difficulty in swallowing liquids, use a straw. This will help the liquids go straight to the esophagus, avoiding painful sores.

In my case, what helped me was mouth washing with organic coconut oil or "swirling". The beneficial antimicrobial properties of coconut oil are long known. Lauric acid in the coconut oil combats bacterial growth in the mouth. The swirling of a small teaspoonful of coconut oil in your mouth for 10 to 15 minutes every morning before breakfast or brushing your teeth works wonders. It also lines your mouth protecting it from damage. During chemo, I would do this several times a day, keeping my mouth moist. Also, keep a glass of water close to you, and continually sip water; maintaining your mouth moist, will help enormously.

Numbness and tingling. These feelings can appear in your hands and feet. It is called peripheral neuropathy. It is the side effect of some chemo drugs. These damage nerves in your arms and legs. Additional symptoms may appear, such as stabbing pain that comes and goes, burning, muscle weakness, keeping your balance, and inability to feel hot or cold temperatures. Talk to your doctor because no treatment fits all symptoms. There is an easy way to prevent these symptoms, yet your doctor can prescribe acupuncture, massage; Exercise; Medicines, transcutaneous nerve stimulation, or Transcutaneous electrical nerve stimulation (TENS).

SUMMARY

Conventional treatments include:

Radiotherapy or radiation. High-energy particles are focused on the tumor to destroy cancer cells. Usually, an external beam is used. **Brachytherapy** is another way of treatment. It uses a "radioactive seed" that is placed in the tumor or near it. This treatment is usually used to treat prostate cancer. A novel form of oral radiation is also being used, where a radioactive ingredient is orally taken although it can also be injected.

Chemotherapy. It uses drugs to destroy cancerous cells, although these drugs also affect healthy cells. Your Oncologist will decide what drugs are specific for your type of cancer, and how these drugs will be administered. They are usually administered through an intravenous injection, although they can also be administered orally. The cycles of the treatment vary. They can be daily, weekly, or monthly. Sometimes when the patient has a difficult vein location or is sensitive to the drugs used, a Vascular Access is implanted. This consists of an internal (subcutaneous), or external port, where the chemotherapy staff will have easy access to introducing and administering the drug.

Hormonal Therapy. In some cases of prostate cancer and **breast cancer**, the cancerous cells are stimulated in their growth by hormones in our bodies. The objective of these treatments is to control these hormones, namely estrogen, and testosterone, and stop them from stimulating cancer cells.

Biological Therapy or Immunotherapy. This treatment aims to stimulate the immune system in our bodies to identify and attack cancerous cells.

Surgery. The option of surgery is not for everybody, as in many cases the simple use of radiation and chemotherapy is enough to eradicate the tumor. Only about 67% of cancer patients will have this option.

Recent development in treatments. The science to combat cancer is moving quickly, and there are new methods of treating types of cancer that surface every day. You should talk to your doctor about this to see if this can be an option for you. New immunotherapies, tumor starvation treatments, and targeted cancer treatments. All these are described in the preceding chapter.

Clinical trials. I make a special mention of these activities that are being conducted by serious institutions all over the country. Their sole aim is to improve existing and approved treatments, and most importantly to improve the quality of life of cancer patients. Please talk to your doctor to see if your type of cancer can take part in these programs.

Side effects of treatment.

As I mentioned before, radiation and chemotherapy not only attack cancerous cells, but they also affect healthy cells, creating side effects that should be monitored. These are some of the most common side effects.

- Hair Loss
- Fatigue
- Nausea
- Pain
- Flu-like symptoms
- Itching
- Mouth sores
- Tingling on hands and feet.

All these should immediately be discussed with your doctor, as the severity of these should be controlled by medication.

CHAPTER FIVE

"There is no greater danger than underestimating your opponent".
— **Lao Tzu**

BREAST CANCER

Breast cancer is a malignancy that originates in the breast. It can originate in either breast. This happens when cells in the breast start to multiply without control at an accelerated speed. This happens because of faulty DNA replication and the faulty cells are not discarded by the auto-defense mechanisms in our body.

Breast cancer almost exclusively affects women, yet there are cases where men can experience this disease.

Some women discover lumps in their breasts during self-examination and immediately think of cancer. It is essential to realize that the majority of breast lumps are benign and not cancer. Noncancerous breast tumors are abnormal growths that do not extend beyond the breast. Any breast lump or change should be evaluated by a medical professional to determine whether it is benign or malignant and whether it may impact your future cancer risk.

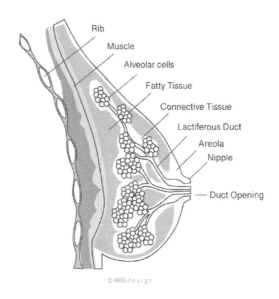

© MUG design

BENIGN TUMORS

Although technically, any lump formed by body cells is referred to as a tumor. Not all tumors are cancerous. The majority of breast lumps (80% of those biopsied) are benign (non-cancerous). The following are some of the most common benign breast conditions that cause lumps.

Changes in fibrocystic tissue:

This is not a disease, but rather a benign (non-cancerous) condition that affects 50-60% of all women. Fibrous breast tissue, mammary glands, and ducts overreact to normal ovulation hormones, resulting in the formation of fibrous lumps and/or numerous, small multiple cysts (lumpy, fluid-filled sacs, or "pockets"). Fibrocystic changes are an exaggerated response of breast tissue to ovarian hormone fluctuations.

The most common non-cancerous breast condition is fibrocystic changes. Women between the ages of 20 and 50 are the most susceptible. Unless a woman is taking hormones, they are unusual after menopause.

Fibrocystic lumps typically grow larger before menstruation and shrink after the period is over. After menopause, this condition, also known as cystic mastitis, usually goes away. There is still disagreement among doctors about whether Fibrocystic disease increases the risk of breast cancer.

According to recent research, the chemical methylxanthine, which is found in coffee, tea, cola, chocolate, and some diet and cold medications, appears to promote the growth of fibrocystic lumps. In one study, more than half of the women who eliminated the above foods from their diet saw their cysts gradually disappear.

Fibroadenomas:

These benign tumors are fibrous and glandular tissue lumps that form in the lobules. They are most common in women aged 18 to 35 and account for nearly all breast tumors in women under the age of 25. Fibroadenomas are usually not tender (though tenderness may be felt just before menstruation) and are easily palpable. In most cases no treatment is necessary, yet it is always good to let your doctor know that you have a lump in the breast.

Papilloma:

A wart-like lump that forms in one or more of the milk ducts in the breast is known as an intraductal papilloma. It is commonly located near the nipple however, it can also be found elsewhere in the breast. It is a non-cancerous breast disease and most frequent in women over the age of 40 and normally develops on its own as the breast matures.

Men can have intraductal papilloma, but it is quite rare.

The symptoms are when you notice a small lump near the nipple or a discharge of clear or blood-stained fluid from the nipple.

It is sometimes confused with cancer, but it is usually benign. In extreme cases, it will have to be removed surgically.

Breast Cancer Symptoms

Understanding how your breasts normally appear and feel is vital to your breast health. Although routine breast cancer screenings are essential, mammograms do not detect all breast cancers. Consequently, you must know how your breasts ordinarily look and feel, so you can detect any changes in your breasts.

The most prevalent breast cancer symptom is a new tumor or mass. However, breast cancers can also be soft, round, tender, and even painful.

Other probable breast cancer symptoms include:

- Total or partial breast enlargement (even if no lump is felt)
- Skin dimpling (sometimes looking like an orange peel)
- Breast or nipple discomfort • Retraction of the nipple (turning inward)
- Red, desiccated, flaking, or thickened nipple or breast skin • Nipple discharge (other than breast milk)
- Lymph nodes swollen under the arm or close to the collarbone (Sometimes this can be a sign of breast cancer spread even before the original tumor in the breast is large enough to be felt.)

Several of these symptoms can also be brought on by benign (noncancerous) breast conditions. Nonetheless, it is essential to have any new breast mass, tumor, or other change evaluated by an experienced healthcare professional to identify and, if necessary, treat the underlying cause.

Remember that knowing what to look for does not replace having routine breast cancer screenings. Mammography screening can often detect breast cancer before the onset of symptoms. Early detection of breast cancer increases the likelihood of successful treatment.

TYPES OF BREAST CANCER

There exists a wide variety of breast cancer types, which are determined based on the particular cells affected within the breast. Carcinomas are the most common form, with Ductal Carcinoma In Situ (DCIS) and Invasive Ductal Carcinoma being the prominent types known as adenocarcinomas. These cancers originate in the gland cells found in the milk ducts or lobules (milk-producing glands). It's worth noting that certain other cancer types, like angiosarcoma or sarcoma, may develop in the breast, but they are not considered breast cancer since they originate from different breast cells.

Breast cancers are further categorized according to specific proteins or genes that may be present in each cancer. Following a biopsy, tests are conducted on breast cancer cells to identify the presence of estrogen receptors, progesterone receptors, and the HER2 gene or protein. Additionally, the lab carefully examines tumor cells to determine their grade. The combination of specific proteins and tumor grade plays a crucial role in determining the cancer stage and guiding appropriate treatment options

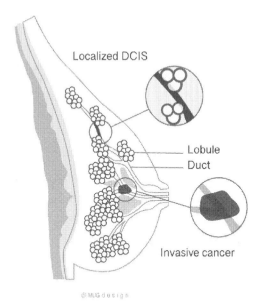

Localized DCIS

Lobule
Duct

Invasive cancer

DIAGNOSIS

Early Breast Cancer Detection

Detecting breast cancer early and receiving cutting-edge cancer treatment are two of the most essential methods for preventing breast cancer complications. Early detection of breast cancer, when it is small and has not spread, makes it simpler to treat successfully. Regular screening is the most effective method to detect breast cancer early.

What are diagnostic screenings?

Screening refers to tests and examinations used to detect a disease in asymptomatic individuals. The purpose of breast cancer screening examinations is to detect the disease early before symptoms appear. (Like a lump in the breast that can be felt). Early detection is the process of discovering and diagnosing a disease before the onset of symptoms.

During screening examinations, breast cancers are more likely to be smaller and less likely to have spread beyond the breast. The extent to which breast cancer has spread, and its magnitude, are two of the most influential factors in determining a woman's outlook on this disease.

- The screening parameters for breast cancer are recommended for women considered at high risk due to factors such as a personal history of breast cancer, a significant family history of breast cancer, or the presence of a genetic mutation associated with increased breast cancer risk (e.g., in a BRCA gene). Additionally, if a woman has undergone chest radiation therapy before the age of 30, she is also considered to be at high risk for breast cancer. For these women the following screening parameters are recommended:
- Women between the ages of 40 and 44 have the option to begin annual mammogram screenings.
- Women 45 to 54 should have annual mammograms.
- Women 55 and older can transition to every other year mammograms or continue with annual

mammograms. Continue screening as long as a woman is in excellent health and is expected to live at least 10 more years.

Breast cancer screening through clinical breast examinations is not recommended for women at moderate risk of breast cancer, regardless of their age. Instead, women in this category should consult their doctors to determine the appropriate screening protocol for their individual needs.

Mammograms

Mammograms are breast X-rays with a low radiation dosage. Regular mammograms can help discover breast cancer early when therapy is most likely to be effective. Typically, a mammogram can detect breast alterations that may be cancerous, years before physical symptoms appear. Several decades of research have proven that women who have regular mammograms are more likely to have breast cancer discovered earlier; requiring fewer severe treatments such as surgery and chemotherapy and are more likely to be cured.

Mammograms are not without flaws. They overlook some cases of breast cancer. And if something is discovered on a screening mammogram, a woman will likely require additional tests such as additional mammograms or a breast ultrasound, to determine whether or not it is cancer. In addition, there is a small possibility of being diagnosed with cancer that would have caused no issues had it not been discovered during screening. It is essential that women who receive mammograms comprehend what to expect and the benefits and limitations of screening.

2D vs. 3D mammography

Digital breast tomosynthesis (commonly known as three-dimensional [3D] mammography) has become increasingly popular in recent years, although it is not available at all breast imaging centers.

Notably, 3D mammograms typically cost more than 2D mammograms, and this additional expense may not be covered by insurance.

Many research studies have shown that 3D mammography seems to lower the chance of needing further tests after initial screening. It also seems to be better at detecting breast cancer, especially in women with dense breasts. Currently, there is a significant ongoing study comparing the results of 3D mammograms with conventional (2D) mammograms.

According to the American Cancer Society (ACS) breast cancer screening guidelines, having a 2D or 3D mammogram is consistent with current screening recommendations. The American Cancer Society also believes that women should be able to choose between 2D and 3D mammography if they or their physician believe that one is more appropriate and that out-of-pocket costs should not be a barrier to having either one.

Clinical breast exam (CBE) and self-exam of the breast (BSE)

Scientific studies indicate that regular breast exams, whether performed by a healthcare professional (clinical breast exams) or by women themselves (self-breast exams), do not offer significant benefits. When combined with mammograms, there is limited evidence that these exams help in detecting breast cancer early. In most cases, breast cancer symptoms, like a breast lump, are discovered by women during everyday activities like bathing or dressing. Therefore, women should be familiar with the look and feel of their breasts and promptly report any changes to a healthcare provider.

Although the American Cancer Society does not recommend routine clinical breast exams or breast self-examinations as part of a breast cancer screening schedule, this does not imply that these exams should never be performed. In certain instances, particularly for women at higher-than-average risk, for instance, health care providers may continue to offer clinical breast evaluations in addition to counseling regarding risk and early detection. Some women may still feel more secure performing regular self-exams to monitor the appearance and texture of their breasts.

American Cancer Society screening guidelines for high-risk women

Women who are at high risk for breast cancer due to certain risk factors should receive a breast MRI and a mammogram annually, beginning at age 30. Also, women that have the following history:

- Have a lifetime risk of breast cancer of 20% to 25% or higher.
- Have a known mutation in the BRCA1 or BRCA2 gene (based on having had genetic testing).
- Have a first-degree relative (parent, sibling, or child) with a BRCA1 or BRCA2 gene mutation and have not themselves undergone genetic testing.
- Received thoracic radiation therapy between 10 and 30 years of age.
- Possess Li-Fraumeni syndrome, Cowden syndrome, or Bannayan-Riley-Ruvalcaba syndrome, or have a first-degree relative with one of these disorders.

The American Cancer Society discourages MRI screening for women with a lifetime breast cancer risk of less than 15%.

There is insufficient evidence to make a recommendation for or against annual MRI screening for women with a higher lifetime risk due to certain factors, such as:

- Having a personal history of breast cancer, ductal carcinoma in situ (DCIS), lobular carcinoma in situ (LCIS), atypical ductal hyperplasia (ADH), or atypical lobular hyperplasia (ALH).

- Having "extremely" or "heterogeneously" dense breasts.

If MRI is used, it should be in addition to a screening mammogram, not in place of one. Even though an MRI is more likely to detect cancer than a mammogram, it may miss some cancer that a mammogram would detect.

The majority of high-risk women should begin screening with MRI and mammograms at age 30 and continue for as long as they remain healthy. However, this decision should be made in consultation with a woman's health care providers, considering her circumstances and preferences into account.

Methods for assessing breast cancer risk.

Several risk assessment tools can assist health professionals in estimating the breast cancer risk of a woman. These tools give rough estimates of breast cancer risk, based on various combinations of risk factors and different data sets. The most common, The Gail Model uses personal medical and reproductive history and family history.

Because each instrument uses different factors to estimate risk, they may yield varying risk estimates for the same woman. Additionally, a woman's risk estimates can change over time.

SCREENING METHODS

Mammograms

Mammograms are low-dose X-rays that can assist in the detection of breast cancer. If you've been told you need a mammogram or are ready to begin breast cancer screening, the following information will help you understand what to expect.

Understanding your performance.

The Breast Imaging Reporting and Data System (BI-RADS) is a standard system used by physicians to characterize what they observe on a mammogram. Learn how to interpret your mammogram results and what it means if they reveal dense breast tissue. Ask your doctor about:

- Mammogram Report Interpretation.
- Breast Density and Your Mammogram Report.
- Mammogram Limitations.

Mammograms in exceptional cases.

If you have had breast cancer in the past, the need to continue receiving mammograms may depend on the type of treatment you received.

If you have breast implants, you can and should receive recommended mammograms. However, the doctor may require additional images to see as much breast tissue as feasible.

Ultrasound of the Breast.

Ultrasound of the breast employs sound waves and their echoes to create computer images of the interior of the breast.

It can detect breast abnormalities, such as fluid-filled cysts, that are more difficult to detect on mammograms.

How is an ultrasound performed?

Ultrasound is not commonly used for regular breast cancer screening. However, it can help to examine breast changes like lumps, especially those that can be felt but not seen on a mammogram. It is particularly beneficial for women with dense breast tissue, which can make it hard for mammograms to detect abnormal areas.

One of the advantages of ultrasound is its ability to distinguish between fluid-filled masses (cysts), which are usually not cancerous, and solid masses that might need further testing to rule out cancer.

Moreover, ultrasound can aid in guiding a biopsy probe to extract cells for cancer testing in the breast or enlarged lymph nodes under the arm. It is a widely available, straightforward procedure that doesn't expose the patient to radiation and is typically more cost-effective than other diagnostic   options.

Ultrasound is a common medical procedure that involves using a handheld device called a transducer. First, a gel is applied to the skin or the transducer, and then the transducer is moved over the skin. It emits sound waves, which bounce back when they encounter body tissues beneath the skin's surface. These echoes are used to create a computer-generated image.

Automated breast ultrasound (ABUS) is a specialized type of ultrasound available at certain imaging facilities. It uses a larger transducer to capture numerous images of the entire breast. ABUS is sometimes used as an extra screening method for women with dense breasts or for those who have abnormal results from other imaging tests or breast-related symptoms. In some cases, a second handheld ultrasound may also be necessary to get more images of suspicious areas.

How are ultrasound breast results reported?

Doctors use the BI-RADS (Breast Imaging Reporting and Data System) to assess mammograms, breast ultrasounds, and breast MRIs. This system categorizes the results from 0 to 6. Using these categories, doctors can easily communicate and describe the findings of an ultrasound, which simplifies discussions about test results and follow-up actions.

Magnetic resonance imaging of the breast.

MRI (magnetic resonance imaging) of the breast uses radio waves and powerful magnets to create detailed images of the breast's interior.

MRI of the breast may be utilized in various situations.

To detect breast cancer, some women at high risk are prescribed an annual mammogram, and in addition, a screening breast MRI. However, the MRI should not be used as a standalone screening test because it may miss some cancer that a mammogram would detect.

While an MRI can detect certain cancer that mammography might miss, it is more prone to detecting non-cancerous findings (false positives). This could lead to unnecessary exams and biopsies for some women. As a result, breast MRI is not recommended as a screening test for women at intermediate risk.

When there are symptoms that could indicate breast cancer, such as suspicious nipple discharge, a breast MRI may be performed, though mammograms and breast ultrasounds are typically conducted first. The MRI is used if the results of these initial tests are inconclusive.

In cases where breast cancer has already been diagnosed, a breast MRI may be performed to precisely determine the size and location of the cancer, look for additional tumors in the breast, and examine the other breast for tumors. However, not every woman with a breast cancer diagnosis requires this test as it may not always be useful.

For screening for implant leaks in women with silicone breast implants, a breast MRI is used. However, this does not apply to women with saline breast implants.

What you need to know about MRIs of the breast.
Breast MRI, like mammograms, needs specialized equipment. The MRI machine used for breast imaging has a unique breast coil. However, not all hospitals and imaging centers possess these specialized MRI machines for breasts. It is essential to have a breast MRI at a facility equipped with dedicated equipment and the capability to perform an MRI-

guided breast biopsy if needed or have a partnership with a facility that can do so.

Unlike using radiation, MRI utilizes powerful magnets to produce highly detailed cross-sectional images of the body. The MRI scanner captures images from various perspectives, resembling how one would observe a segment of your body from the front, side, and above your head. This imaging technique can reveal soft tissue body components that might be difficult to see with other methods.

Unlike mammograms and breast ultrasounds, breast MRI requires the injection of a contrast dye into your vein through an IV line before obtaining the images. This simplifies the detection of any breast abnormalities.

Preparing for the examination.

Check with your insurance company before obtaining an MRI: Before a breast MRI can be performed, your insurance company may need to confirm the expense. The majority of private insurance plans that cover mammogram screening also cover MRI screening if a woman is determined to be at elevated risk. Going to a center with a breast health or high-risk clinic where the staff has experience obtaining approval for breast MRIs may be beneficial.

Breast MRIs are typically performed while the patient is reclining on their stomach with their arms above their head inside a long, narrow tube. If you are uncomfortable in confined spaces, you may need to take medication to help you calm down while in the scanner. Before the test, speaking with the technologist, or a patient counselor, or receiving a tour of the MRI machine can also be beneficial. During the assessment, you will be alone in the exam room, but you can communicate with the MR technologist, who can see and hear what is happening.

Remove metal objects: Before the examination, you will be required to disrobe and don a gown or other non-metallic garments. Remove any metal hair attachments, jewelry, dental work, or body piercings that you can.

If metal is present in your body: The technologist will ask if you have any metal in your body prior to the scan. Some metallic objects are not problematic, while others are.

Inform your technician if your body contains any medical implants or attachments. If you have any of the following types of medical implants, you should not enter the MRI scanning area unless a radiologist or technologist permits you to do so:

- An implanted defibrillator or pacemaker
- Brain aneurysm clips
- A cochlear (ear) implant
- Metal filaments inside blood vessels

Breast MRI.

MRI examinations are typically performed in an outpatient hospital or clinic setting. An IV line will be inserted in your arm to inject a contrast material during the procedure.

You will recline face down on a slender, flat table with your arms extended above your head. Your breasts will dangle through an opening in the table to be scanned without compression. The technician may use cushions to make you comfortable and prevent movement. The table is subsequently slid into a long, thin tube.

The examination is painless, but you need to remain still inside a narrow tube. At certain points, you might be asked to hold your breath or stay motionless. The machine will produce loud thumping, clicking, and whirring sounds, similar to a washing machine, as the magnet turns on and off. Some places might offer earplugs or headphones to reduce the noise.

During a breast MRI to detect breast cancer, they inject a contrast material called gadolinium into a vein in your arm. This material helps highlight any abnormal breast tissue. If you have any allergies to contrast agents or dyes used in imaging tests or had previous issues with them, inform the technologist.

Remaining motionless during the test is crucial for obtaining high-quality images. Each image set usually takes a few minutes, resulting in a total test duration of 30 to 45 minutes. After the test, you might need to wait for the evaluation of the photos to see if additional images are needed.

Abbreviated breast MRI, a newer technique, requires fewer images, reducing the scan time to around 10 minutes.

How are the results of a breast MRI reported?

Physicians utilize a uniform system called BI-RADS (Breast Imaging Reporting and Data System) to assess mammograms, breast ultrasound, and breast MRI results. This system categorizes the findings into numbered groups ranging from 0 to 6. By doing so, doctors can use consistent language to convey the outcomes of a breast MRI, which improves communication about the test results and any necessary follow-up.

Nuclear diagnostics (radionuclide imaging)

A small amount of radioactive material called a tracer, is introduced into the bloodstream for these tests. Cancer cells tend to gather the tracer more than regular cells. A specialized camera is then used to locate the tracer in the breast or other parts of the body.

For molecular breast imaging (MBI), also known as scintimammography or breast-specific gamma imaging (BSGI), a tracer called technetium-99m sestamibi is injected into the bloodstream, and a special camera is used to observe the tracer while gently compressing the breast. This test is primarily being studied to monitor breast issues like lumps or abnormal mammograms or to determine the extent of previously diagnosed breast cancer. It is also being explored as a cancer screening test for women with dense breasts. However, due to potential radiation exposure to the whole body, it is unlikely to be used annually for screening purposes.

In positron emission tomography (PET) scanning, blood is injected with a different radioactive tracer. When there is suspicion that breast cancer has spread to other areas of the body, standard PET scans using radioactive sugar (FDG) are sometimes performed. A newer tracer called Fluoroestradiol F-18 is now available to detect the spread of certain advanced estrogen receptor (ER)-positive breast cancers.

Positron emission mammography (PEM) is a novel breast imaging technique that combines elements of PET scans and mammograms. Both PET and PEM use the same radioactive tracer injected into the bloodstream. The breast is lightly compressed during imaging, similar to a mammogram. PEM may be more effective than standard mammography in detecting small concentrations of breast cancer cells because it considers the activity level of the breast cells, not just their structure. PEM is primarily being researched in women with breast cancer to determine if it can help assess the extent of cancer. However, since PEM exposes the entire body to radiation, it is unlikely to be used annually for breast cancer screening.

Mammography enhanced with contrast (CEM)

This is a new type of test called Contrast-Enhanced Spectral Mammography (CESM). In this test, a special dye with iodine is injected into the bloodstream a few minutes before taking two sets of mammograms using different energy levels. The dye helps the X-rays to better detect abnormal breast tissue. This test is useful for getting a closer look at areas that appear unusual on a regular mammogram or for determining the size of a tumor in women who have recently been diagnosed with breast cancer.

Researchers are currently comparing CESM to breast MRI in these situations, especially when an MRI cannot be done for some reason. They are also considering using CESM to screen women with dense breasts. If CESM proves to be as effective as MRI, it could become more widely used because it is faster and less expensive.

Elastography

This examination is performed as part of an ultrasound exam. It is founded on the notion that breast cancer tumors are typically firmer and stiffer than the surrounding breast tissue. For this technique, the breast is gently compressed, and the ultrasound can reveal the firmness of a suspicious area. This test may be useful in determining whether a suspicious area is malignant or benign.

Optical Imaging procedures

These tests assess the amount of light that returns from or passes through the breast tissue. The technique does not use radiation and does not require breast compression. Combining optical imaging with other tests such as MRI, ultrasound, or 3D mammography to detect breast cancer is the subject of preliminary research.

Electrical Impedance Tomography (EIT)

EIT is predicated on the premise that breast cancer cells conduct electricity differently than healthy cells. For this test, very tiny electrical currents are passed through the breast and detected on the skin using small electrodes adhered to the skin. EIT does not utilize radiation or breast compression. This test may prove beneficial in helping to classify mammogram-detected tumors. However, not enough clinical testing has been conducted to determine if it is beneficial for breast cancer screening.

TREATMENTS

Surgical treatment for breast cancer

The majority of women with breast cancer undergo surgery as part of their treatment. Depending on the circumstances, various types of breast surgery may be performed for different reasons. For instance, surgery may be performed to:

- Remove as much cancer as possible.
- Determine if the cancer has spread to the lymph nodes in the armpit.
- Restore the contour of the breast after cancer removal.
- Relieve advanced cancer symptoms

Your doctor may recommend a specific surgery based on the characteristics of your breast cancer and your medical history, or you may have a choice regarding the type of surgery to undergo. It is essential to understand your options so that you can discuss them with your doctor and make an informed decision.

Surgical removal of breast carcinoma

There are two main types of surgeries to remove breast cancer: mastectomy and lumpectomy. In lumpectomy (also known as quadrantectomy, partial mastectomy, or segmental mastectomy), only the cancerous portion of the breast and some surrounding normal tissue are removed, depending on the tumor's location, size, and other factors.

On the other hand, mastectomy involves the complete removal of the entire breast, along with all breast tissue and sometimes nearby tissues as well. There are different types of mastectomies, and some women may opt for a double mastectomy, where both breasts are removed.

Breast-conserving surgery (BCS) and mastectomy are options for women with early-stage breast cancer. BCS allows women to keep most of their breasts but usually requires radiation. On the other hand, women who choose mastectomy for early-stage cancer are less likely to need radiation.

Mastectomy might be the best or only choice for some women based on the type of breast cancer, tumor size, previous radiation, and other factors.

Some women worry that choosing a less invasive surgery like BCS may increase the risk of cancer recurrence. However, extensive studies spanning more than two decades show that when BCS is combined with radiation, the outlook is similar to that of mastectomy for early-stage cancer patients eligible for both procedures.

To determine the stage of breast cancer and whether it has spread to the underarm lymph nodes, some of these nodes will be removed and examined in the laboratory. This step is crucial in assessing the cancer's size and spread.

There are two main types of lymph node removal surgeries:

- Sentinel lymph node biopsy (SLNB): In this procedure, a dye is injected under the arm, and only the lymph nodes that absorb the dye are removed. These nodes are likely to be the first ones affected by cancer spread. Removing only a few nodes reduces the risk of complications like lymphedema (arm swelling).

- Axillary lymph node dissection (ALND): In ALND, the surgeon removes several (usually fewer than 20) underarm lymph nodes without the use of a dye. Although performed less frequently nowadays, ALND may still be necessary in specific situations to examine the lymph nodes thoroughly.

Wire localization to guide surgery

If breast cancer cannot be felt, is hard to find, or is difficult to reach, a surgeon may use a mammogram or ultrasound to guide a wire to the right location in a procedure called wire or needle localization. A local anesthetic is used to numb the breast, and a thin, hollow needle is guided to the abnormal area. Once properly positioned, a thin wire with a hook at the end is inserted through the needle and left in place as a guide. In the operating room, the wire helps the surgeon locate the portion of the breast to be removed.

This wire localization surgery may be considered breast-conserving if all cancer is removed and margins are clear. However, if cancer cells are found near the removed tissue's edges (positive or close margin), additional surgery may be needed.

The wire-localization procedure is also used for surgical biopsies of suspicious breast areas to determine if they are cancerous.

After breast cancer surgery, many women may consider breast reconstruction to restore the appearance of their breasts. Depending on the circumstances, different types of reconstructive surgery are available, and the timing of reconstruction can be immediate or delayed. It's important to discuss these options with both the breast surgeon and a plastic surgeon before the main cancer surgery to determine the best approach.

In cases of advanced breast cancer that has spread to other parts of the body, surgery may not cure the cancer, but it can be beneficial in certain situations. Surgery may be used to slow the cancer's spread, alleviate symptoms, treat specific areas with limited cancer spread, or relieve pressure on organs or bones caused by the cancer.

If surgery is recommended for advanced breast cancer, it's crucial to understand whether the goal is to cure the cancer or to manage symptoms.

Radiation treatment for breast cancer

Radiation therapy is the destruction of cancer cells by high-energy radiation (or particles). In addition to other therapies, some women with breast cancer will need radiation.

Depending on the stage of the breast cancer and other factors, radiation therapy may be used in a variety of situations:

- Following breast-conserving surgery (BCS), to reduce the likelihood of cancer recurring in the same breast or adjacent lymph nodes.
- Following a mastectomy, particularly if the cancer was larger than 5 centimeters (approximately 2 inches) if it is found in numerous lymph nodes, or if certain surgical margins, such as skin or muscle, contain cancer cells.
- If the malignancy has spread to other organs, such as the bones, spinal cord, or brain.

Types of Radiation therapy

The primary methods of radiation therapy employed for breast cancer treatment are external beam radiation and brachytherapy.

External radiation beam therapy (EBRT)

EBRT, the most common radiation therapy for breast cancer, uses an external machine to target the cancerous area. Whether you need radiation treatment depends on whether you had a mastectomy or breast-conserving surgery and if the cancer has spread to nearby lymph nodes.

Here are the scenarios for radiation treatment:

Mastectomy without cancerous lymph nodes: Radiation focuses on the chest wall, mastectomy scar, and drainage exit points after surgery.

Breast-conserving surgery (BCS): The whole breast is usually irradiated (whole breast radiation). If there's a high risk of cancer recurrence, the area where the cancer was removed (tumor bed) may also receive additional radiation after the full breast treatment. This additional radiation (boost radiation) is given with lower intensity and typically after the main breast treatment. The majority of women do not notice different side effects between boost radiation and whole breast radiation.

If cancer is found in the lymph nodes under the arm (axillary lymph nodes), radiation may be applied to this area. In some cases, radiation may also include the lymph nodes above the collarbone (supraclavicular lymph nodes) and beneath the breastbone in the middle of the chest (internal mammary lymph nodes).

If you require external beam radiation therapy after surgery, it usually begins at least a month after your surgery site has healed. If you're undergoing chemotherapy, radiation treatments are usually delayed until after chemotherapy is completed. Radiation can be given together with hormone therapy or HER2-targeted therapy, if applicable, after surgery.

Radiation Procedures.

Total breast radiotherapy: This involves radiation to the entire affected breast. The standard schedule is 5 days per week (Monday to Friday) for about 6 to 7 weeks.

Another option is hypofractionated radiation therapy, where larger daily doses are given (Monday to Friday) but with fewer treatments, usually 3 to 4 weeks. Studies have shown that this shorter schedule is as effective in preventing cancer recurrence in the same breast for women who had breast-conserving surgery and no cancer spread to underarm lymph nodes. It may also result in fewer short-term side effects.

Accelerated Partial Breast Irradiation.

After undergoing whole breast radiation therapy or surgery alone, most breast cancers tend to come back near the area where the tumor was removed, called the tumor bed. To address this, some doctors use accelerated partial breast irradiation (APBI). This involves delivering higher doses of radiation to only the tumor bed over a shorter time instead of treating the entire breast, but its long-term effectiveness compared to conventional radiation is still being studied, so not all doctors use it. There are several types of accelerated partial breast irradiation:

Intraoperative radiation therapy (IORT): This method delivers a significant dose of radiation to the tumor bed immediately after breast-conserving surgery (BCS) and before closing the incision. It requires specialized equipment that is not widely available.

3D-conformal radiotherapy (3D-CRT): In this technique, specialized devices are used to target the tumor bed more precisely, preserving more of the normal surrounding breast tissue. Treatments are given twice daily for five days or every day for two weeks.

Intensity-modulated radiotherapy (IMRT): Similar to 3D-CRT, IMRT adjusts the intensity of specific radiation beams. This allows higher doses to be delivered to specific areas of the tumor bed while minimizing damage to nearby healthy tissues.

Brachytherapy: Brachytherapy administers radiation therapy precisely to the internal location of breast cancer cells. This technique entails the insertion of a radioactive source into the surgical site following the removal of a breast lump by the surgeon. The radiation is limited to a small area surrounding the surgical site exclusively.

Women interested in these methods can discuss participating in accelerated partial breast irradiation clinical trials with their physicians.

For those who have had a mastectomy and have no affected lymph nodes, radiation is administered to the entire chest wall, the mastectomy scar, and any surgical drain sites. This treatment is typically given daily, five days a week, for six weeks.

Radiotherapy in lymph nodes

If cancer was detected in the lymph nodes under the arm (axillary lymph nodes), radiation may be administered, regardless of whether BCS or a mastectomy has been performed. In some instances, the lymph nodes above the clavicle (supraclavicular lymph nodes) and behind the breastbone in the center of the chest (internal mammary lymph nodes) will also receive radiation alongside the underarm lymph nodes. It is typically administered daily, five days per week, for six weeks concurrently with radiation to the breast or chest wall.

Possible External Beam Radiation adverse effects

The primary short-term adverse effects of breast external beam radiation therapy are:

- Breast swelling.
- Sunburn-like skin changes in the treated area (redness, peeling, discoloration of the skin)
- Fatigue.

- Your health care team may advise you to avoid sun exposure on the treated skin, as it could exacerbate the skin changes. The majority of skin alterations improve within a few months. Usually, breast tissue changes disappear within six to twelve months, but it may take longer.

- Later on, external beam radiation therapy can also induce the following side effects:

- Radiation therapy may cause some women's breasts to shrink and their epidermis to become firmer or swollen.

- Radiation can impact your choices for breast reconstruction in the future. It may also raise the likelihood of appearance and healing issues, especially when administered after reconstruction, specifically with tissue flap procedures.

- Women who have undergone breast radiation may be unable to breastfeed from the radiated breast. This condition is known as brachial plexopathy and can cause tingling, pain, and paralysis in the shoulder, arm, and hand.

- Lymphedema, a condition that causes pain and swelling in the arm or torso, may be caused by lymph node radiation to the underarm. In rare instances, radiation therapy may weaken the ribs, which could lead to a fracture.

- In the past, women were more likely to receive radiation to the lungs and heart, which could cause long-term injury to these organs. Modern radiation therapy equipment focuses the radiation beams more precisely than older devices; therefore, these issues are uncommon today. An angiosarcoma is a very rare complication of radiation therapy to the breast.

If you have any apprehension about radiation side effects, you should discuss them with your doctor. It is important to note that I name all possibilities, yet they are not the norm.

Brachytherapy

Brachytherapy, also referred to as internal radiation, is another method of administering radiation therapy. Instead of directing radiation beams from outside the body, a device containing radioactive seeds or pellets is inserted into the breast tissue in the area where the cancer had been excised for a brief period. (Tumor bed).

As a form of accelerated partial breast irradiation, brachytherapy can be used alone (instead of radiation to the entire breast) for certain women who have undergone breast-conserving surgery (BCS). Who can receive brachytherapy may be restricted by tumor size, location, and other factors.

Variations on brachytherapy

Intracavitary Radiation Therapy

This is the most common form of brachytherapy for breast cancer patients. A device is inserted into the space left by BCS and left in place until treatment is complete. There are numerous available devices, the majority of which need surgical training for appropriate placement. They are all inserted as a thin catheter into the breast. The end of the device placed within the breast is then expanded like a balloon to ensure that it remains securely in position throughout the treatment. The opposite extremity of the catheter protrudes from the breast. For each procedure, one or more sources of radiation (often pellets) are inserted down the tube and into the device for a brief period before being removed. Typically, treatments are administered twice daily for five days in an ambulatory setting. Following the conclusion of the last treatment, the device is deflated and removed.

Interstitial Radiation Therapy

Several catheters are inserted into the breast and left in position for several days around the area where the cancer was removed. Daily, the catheters are implanted with radioactive pellets for brief periods and then removed. This method of brachytherapy has been around longer (and is supported by more evidence), but it is not as popular.

Early studies of intracavitary brachytherapy as the only radiation after BCS have shown promising results in terms of achieving at least the same level of cancer control as standard whole breast radiation, but there may be more complications, such as poor cosmetic outcomes. This treatment is currently the subject of research, and more follow-up is required.

Possible Intracavitary Brachytherapy adverse consequences

As with external beam radiation, intracavitary brachytherapy can cause side effects, such as:

- Redness and/or bruising at the treatment site
- Breast pain
- Infection
- Damage to fatty tissue in the breast
- In uncommon cases, weakness and rib fracture
- Fluid accumulation within the breast (seroma)
- Additional information on radiation therapy

Systemic therapies

Because they can reach cancer cells almost everywhere in the body, drugs used to treat breast cancer are categorized as systemic therapies. Some can be administered orally, via muscle injection, or directly into the circulation. Depending on the form of breast cancer, the following drug treatments may be administered:

Treatment with chemotherapy for breast cancer

Chemotherapy (chemo) employs anti-cancer medicines that may be administered intravenously (into a vein) or orally. The medications travel through the bloodstream to reach cancer cells in the majority of body locations. Occasionally, if cancer has progressed to the spinal fluid that surrounds and cushions the brain and spinal cord, chemotherapy may be administered directly into this area. (Called intrathecal chemotherapy).

Chemotherapy

Chemotherapy is not necessary for all women with breast cancer, but there are several instances in which it may be recommended.

After surgery, (Adjuvant Chemotherapy)

Chemotherapy may be administered to eliminate any cancer cells that may have been left behind or that have spread but cannot be detected by imaging tests. These cells are microscopic because they are not visible to the naked eye. If these cells were permitted to proliferate, they could form cancers elsewhere in the body. Adjuvant chemotherapy can reduce the recurrence risk of breast cancer. After breast surgery, there are tests, such as Oncotype DX, that can help determine which women will most likely benefit from chemotherapy. Gene Expression Tests for Breast Cancer provide additional information.

Before surgery (neoadjuvant chemotherapy)

The goal of neoadjuvant chemotherapy is to reduce the tumor so that it can be removed with less invasive surgery. Consequently, neoadjuvant chemotherapy is frequently used to treat cancers that are too large to be removed by surgery at the time of initial diagnosis, have numerous lymph nodes implicated, or are inflammatory breast cancers.

If, following neoadjuvant chemotherapy, cancer cells are still detected during surgery (also known as residual disease), you may be offered additional chemotherapy (adjuvant chemotherapy) to reduce the likelihood of the cancer returning. (recurrence).

Other reasons you may receive neoadjuvant chemotherapy:

Giving chemotherapy before removing the tumor allows doctors to observe how the cancer responds to the treatment. If the initial chemotherapy doesn't shrink the tumor, the doctor will know that more medications are needed. Additionally, this approach can target and eliminate cancer cells that may have spread but are not visible through regular exams or imaging tests. Neoadjuvant chemotherapy, like adjuvant chemotherapy, can lower the risk of breast cancer recurrence. For some people with early-stage cancer, completely eradicating cancer through neoadjuvant chemotherapy may lead to longer survival, especially in cases of triple-negative or HER2-positive breast cancer. Administering chemotherapy before surgery can also offer certain patients more time for genetic testing or planning reconstructive surgery. However, it's important to note that not all breast cancer patients are suitable candidates for neoadjuvant chemotherapy.

For advanced breast cancer

Chemotherapy can be the primary treatment for women whose breast and underarm cancer has progressed to distant organs such as the liver and lungs. Chemotherapy can be administered either at the time of breast cancer diagnosis or after initial treatments. The duration of treatment depends on the efficacy and tolerability of the chemotherapy.

Chemotherapeutic agents used to treat breast cancer

In most instances, chemotherapy is most effective when multiple drugs are administered simultaneously. Frequently, two or three medications are combined. Numerous drug combinations are employed by physicians.

For HER2-positive cancers, one or more medications that target HER2 may be combined with chemotherapy.

How is chemotherapy administered for breast cancer?

Typically, chemotherapy drugs for breast cancer are administered intravenously (IV), either as an injection over a few minutes or as an infusion over a prolonged duration. This can be performed in a hospital, doctor's office, or infusion center.

Frequently, a slightly larger and more robust IV is required to administer chemotherapy through the venous system. These are referred to as central venous catheters, central venous access devices, or central lines. They are utilized to administer medications, blood products, nutrients, or fluids directly into the bloodstream. Additionally, they can be used to draw blood for testing.

There are numerous varieties of CVCs. The port and PICC lines are the most common varieties. For patients with breast cancer, the central line is typically placed on the opposing side of the tumor. If a woman has breast cancer in both breasts, the central line will likely be inserted on the side where fewer lymph nodes were removed or were affected by cancer.

Chemotherapy is administered in cycles, followed by a period of leisure to allow patients to recover from the side effects of the drugs. Chemotherapy regimens typically last two to three weeks. The schedule varies based on the substances used. With certain medications, chemotherapy is administered only on the first day of the cycle. Others receive it once per week or every other week for a few weeks. After the cycle, the chemotherapy regimen is repeated to initiate the next cycle.

On average, adjuvant and neoadjuvant chemotherapy is administered for a total of three to six months, depending on the medicines employed. The duration of treatment for metastatic (Stage 4) breast cancer is dependent on its efficacy and adverse effects.

Concentrated medicines

Doctors have discovered that administering cycles of certain chemotherapy drugs more frequently can reduce the likelihood of cancer recurrence and enhance survival for some breast cancer patients. For instance, a substance that would ordinarily be administered every three weeks could be administered every two weeks. This applies to both neoadjuvant and adjuvant therapy. It can exacerbate low blood cell counts, so it is not an option for every woman.

Possible chemotherapy adverse effects on breast cancer

Chemotherapy drugs can induce side effects, depending on the type, dose, and duration of treatment.

- Hair loss
- Nail changes
- Mouth ulcers
- Appetite loss or weight fluctuations are among the most common potential side effects.
- Nausea and vomiting
- Diarrhea
- Fatigue
- Hot flashes and/or vaginal dryness brought on by menopause and chemotherapy
- Nerve harm
- Chemotherapy can also affect the blood-forming cells in the bone marrow, which can result in:
- A higher risk of infection (from low white blood cell counts)
- Easy bruising or hemorrhaging (from low blood platelet counts)
- Fatigue (from low red blood cell counts and other reasons)

Typically, these adverse effects disappear once treatment is completed. There are frequent methods to mitigate these adverse effects. For instance, medications can be administered to prevent or reduce nausea and vomiting.

Other possible adverse effects also exist. Some of these are more common with specific chemotherapy medications. Inquire with your cancer care team about the potential adverse effects of the drugs you are receiving.

Menstrual fluctuations and fertility concerns

Chemotherapy often leads to changes in menstrual cycles in younger women, which can result in permanent premature menopause and infertility. This may increase the risk of heart disease, bone loss, and osteoporosis. Fortunately, there are drugs available to prevent or treat bone loss.

Even if your periods stop during chemotherapy, it's still possible to become pregnant. However, getting pregnant while undergoing chemotherapy can lead to birth defects and interfere with treatment. If you haven't reached menopause and are sexually active, it's crucial to discuss birth control options with your doctor. Hormonal birth control, like birth control pills, is not recommended for women with hormone receptor-positive breast cancer. Hence, consulting both your oncologist and gynecologist (or family doctor) about suitable options is important. After completing cancer treatment, it is generally safe for women to have children, but getting pregnant during treatment is not advised.

If you wish to have children after breast cancer treatment, it's essential to discuss this with your doctor as early as possible, ideally before starting treatment. Some women may benefit from additional measures, like monthly injections of a luteinizing hormone-releasing hormone (LHRH) analog, to increase the chances of a successful pregnancy after cancer treatment.

Heart injury

Although it is uncommon and a few chemotherapeutic agents can induce irreversible heart damage. (Called cardiomyopathy). The risk is greatest when the drug is used for an extended time or at large doses. Other drugs that can cause heart injury (such as those that target HER2) increase the likelihood of damage from these medications. Other risk factors for heart failure, such as a family history of heart disease, hypertension, and diabetes, can also place you at risk if you take one of these medications.

Before prescribing one of these medications, the majority of physicians will conduct a heart function test, such as an echocardiogram (also known as an ECHO) or a MUGA scan. During treatment, they may also closely monitor for signs of cardiac problems and repeat heart tests regularly. If cardiac function begins to deteriorate, these medications will be temporarily or permanently discontinued. However, in some cases, harm may not manifest until months or years after treatment is discontinued.

Nerve injury (neuropathy)

Some chemotherapy medications can cause nerve injury in the hands, arms, feet, and legs. This may result in symptoms such as numbness, pain, burning or tingling sensations, sensitivity to cold or heat, or fatigue in the affected areas. In the majority of cases, these symptoms disappear once treatment is discontinued.

Hand-foot syndrome

Certain chemotherapy medications can irritate the palms and soles of the hands and feet. It is known as hand-foot syndrome. Among the earliest symptoms are numbness, trembling, and redness. If the condition worsens, the hands and feet may swell and become bothersome or even painful. The epidermis may blister, resulting in peeling or even sores. Although there is no specific treatment, some lotions or steroids administered before chemotherapy may be helpful. These symptoms progressively improve when the drug is discontinued, or the dosage is reduced. The best method to prevent severe hand-foot syndrome is to inform your doctor as soon as symptoms appear so that the drug dose can be adjusted, or other medications can be prescribed.

Chemo mind

Many breast cancer patients who undergo chemotherapy report a modest decline in cognitive function. They may experience concentration and memory issues that persist for an extended time. Nevertheless, the majority of women function well after treatment is over.

Hormones therapy

Certain forms of breast cancer are influenced by estrogen and progesterone. Breast cancer cells contain receptors (proteins) that bind to estrogen and progesterone, thereby promoting their growth. Hormone or endocrine therapy refers to treatments that prevent hormones from attaching to their receptors.

Hormone therapy can target cancer cells virtually everywhere in the body, not just in the breast. It is indicated for women with **hormone receptor-positive** tumors. It is ineffective for women whose cancer lacks hormone receptors.

Typically, it is taken for long periods. Women whose cancer has a higher likelihood of recurrence may be offered treatment lasting longer. A test called the Breast Cancer Index may be used to determine if a woman will benefit from hormone therapy for more than five years.

Hormone therapy can also be used to treat cancer that has recurred or disseminated to other parts of the body after initial treatment.

Approximately two-thirds of breast cancer is hormone receptor-positive. Their cells contain estrogen (ER-positive cancers) and/or progesterone (PR-positive cancers) receptors (proteins) that aid in the growth and spread of cancer cells.

There are numerous hormone therapies for breast cancer. The majority of hormone therapies either reduce estrogen levels or prevent estrogen from promoting the growth of breast cancer cells.

Targeted Treatment

Targeted drug therapy employs drugs that target proteins in breast cancer cells that promote their growth, spread, and survival. Targeted drugs operate to destroy or slow the development of cancer cells, and can be administered intravenously (IV), subcutaneously (SC), or orally (pill).

Some targeted therapy medicines, such as monoclonal antibodies, control cancer cells in multiple ways and may also be considered immunotherapy because they stimulate the immune system.

As with chemotherapy, these medicines enter the bloodstream and reach nearly all areas of the body, making them effective against cancers that have spread to distant organs. Sometimes, targeted medicines work even when chemotherapy does not. Some targeted medications can improve the efficacy of other forms of treatment.

In approximately 15% to 20% of breast cancer, the cells produce an excessive amount of the growth-promoting protein HER2. Known as HER2-positive breast cancers, these cancers tend to grow and disseminate more aggressively than HER2-negative breast cancers.

Antibody-drug conjugates

ADCs are monoclonal antibodies attached to chemotherapy drugs. The anti-HER2 antibody works as a homing signal by binding to the HER2 protein on cancer cells, thereby directing chemotherapeutic agents directly to the cancer cells.

Kinase inhibiting agents.

HER2 is a kinase, a category of protein. Kinases are intracellular proteins that normally transmit signals (such as telling the cell to grow). Inhibitors of kinases are known as kinase inhibitors.

Side effects of HER2 targeted medication

The adverse effects of HER2-targeted medications are typically mild. Discuss your expectations with your doctor. If you are pregnant, you should avoid taking these medications. They can cause damage to the fetus. Discuss effective contraception with your doctor if you could become pregnant while taking these medications.

Occasionally, monoclonal antibodies and antibody-drug conjugates can induce cardiac damage during or following treatment. This can ultimately result in congestive heart failure. For most women, this effect is temporary and improves when the drug is discontinued.

Due to the potential for these drugs to cause cardiac damage, your heart function is frequently evaluated (using an echocardiogram or MUGA scan) before treatment and regularly while you are taking the medication. Notify your doctor if you develop symptoms such as shortness of breath, rapid heart rate, swollen legs, and extreme fatigue.

Targeted therapy for breast cancer with positive hormone receptors

Approximately three out of four breast cancers are hormone receptor-positive (estrogen or progesterone). Hormone therapy is frequently effective in treating these cancers in women. Certain targeted therapy drugs can enhance the efficacy of hormone therapy.

Personalized treatment for females with BRCA gene mutations

Only a small portion of breast cancer patients have a mutated BRCA gene, which exists in all cells of their body. This gene mutation is different from the genetic changes that occur later and are specific to cancer cells. Before starting treatment with these medications, your doctor will check for a BRCA mutation in your blood if it's not already known.

Possible side effects of these medications include low red blood cell counts (anemia), low platelet counts, and low white blood cell counts.

Immunotherapy for the Treatment of Breast Cancer

Immunotherapy is the use of drugs to enhance a patient's immune system's ability to recognize and eliminate cancer cells. Immunotherapy typically enhances the immune response by targeting specific proteins involved in the immune system. These medications have adverse effects distinct from chemotherapy.

Some immunotherapy medicines, such as monoclonal antibodies, control cancer cells in multiple ways and may also be considered targeted therapy because they inhibit the growth of cancer cells by blocking a specific protein.

The immune system's ability to refrain from attacking normal cells in the body is an essential function. To accomplish this, it employs proteins (or "checkpoints") on immune cells that must be activated (or deactivated) to initiate an immune response. Sometimes, breast cancer cells utilize these checkpoints to circumvent immune system attacks. These checkpoint proteins are targeted by drugs that restore the immune response against breast cancer cells.

Possible immune checkpoint inhibitor adverse effects

These medications may cause side effects such as fatigue, cough, vertigo, skin rash, loss of appetite, constipation, and diarrhea.

Some individuals may experience an infusion reaction while receiving these medications. This is similar to an allergic reaction and can include fever, shivers, facial flushing, rash, itchy skin, dizziness, wheezing, and difficulty breathing. It is crucial to inform your doctor or nurse immediately if you experience any of these symptoms while taking these medications.

It is essential to promptly inform your doctor of any new side effects. If severe adverse effects occur, treatment may be discontinued, and you may be given high doses of corticosteroids to suppress the immune system.

BREAST CANCER TREATMENT BY STAGE

The information provided here is based on AJCC Staging systems used before 2018, primarily considering tumor size and lymph node status. However, the updated breast cancer staging system now incorporates additional factors like estrogen receptor (ER), progesterone receptor (PR), and HER2 status. Consequently, this might result in higher or lower stages compared to the previous systems. To make informed decisions about your treatment, it is essential to discuss this with your doctor.

When dealing with breast cancer, determining the stage is crucial in shaping the appropriate treatment options. Generally, the more advanced the cancer, the greater the likelihood of requiring additional treatments. Besides tumor size and lymph node status, other important factors include the presence of hormone receptors (ER-positive or PR-positive) and high levels of the HER2 protein (HER2-positive). Additionally, specific gene mutations and your overall well-being and individual preferences play a role in determining the most suitable treatment plan.

Other considerations include whether you have experienced menopause, the rate at which the cancer is growing and whether it has spread to vital organs like the lungs or liver. All of these variables should be discussed thoroughly with your physician to understand how they might impact your treatment options. Your doctor's care and expertise, combined with open communication about your condition, will guide you toward the most appropriate and personalized approach to managing breast cancer.

STAGE 0

Non-invasive stage 0 cancer refers to a condition where cancer cells are limited to the milk ducts and do not spread to surrounding tissues. At its earliest stage, this type of cancer is known as Ductal Carcinoma in Situ (DCIS) in the breast.

Recently, the classification of lobular carcinoma in situ (LCIS) has been updated, and it is no longer categorized as stage 0 cancer. However, it does signify an elevated risk of developing breast cancer in the future. Lobular Carcinoma in Situ (LCIS) provides additional important information in this regard.

STAGES I TO III

Treatment for breast cancer in stages I to III typically involves a combination of surgery and radiation therapy. In some cases, chemotherapy or other drug therapies may be administered either before the surgery (neoadjuvant) or after the surgery (adjuvant).

Stage I breast cancers are relatively small and may not have spread to the lymph nodes, or if they have, it's only a small area in the sentinel lymph node (the first node at risk of cancer spread).

Stage II breast cancers are larger than stage I and may have spread to a few nearby lymph nodes.

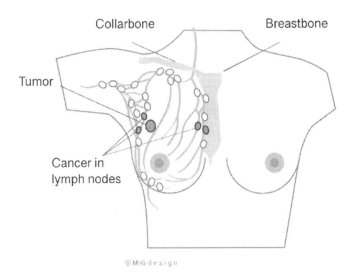

Stage III breast cancers are larger and may be growing into nearby tissues like the skin over the breast or the underlying muscle. Alternatively, they might have spread to multiple nearby lymph nodes.

The stage of breast cancer is a critical factor in determining the appropriate course of treatment. For women diagnosed with breast cancer in stages I, II, or III, treatment typically involves surgery, often followed by radiation therapy. Additionally, systemic drug therapy, which targets cancer cells throughout the body, is commonly employed.

The extent of breast cancer spread plays a significant role in shaping the treatment plan, though individual preferences and specific characteristics of the cancer, such as hormone receptor status, HER2 protein levels, growth rate, overall health, and menopausal status, also influence the treatment options.

In this context, it is important to have a comprehensive discussion with your healthcare provider to explore the various factors that may affect your treatment choices. Among the different drug treatment options available, chemotherapy, hormone therapy, targeted drugs, as well as immunotherapy, are some of the potential systemic therapies considered. The choice of drugs best suited for your case depends on factors like hormone receptor status, HER2 status, and other relevant considerations. By understanding these options, you can work together with your medical team to develop a personalized treatment plan that offers the best chances for successful outcomes.

STAGE IV

In advanced cases of breast cancer, referred to as Stage IV, the cancer cells have extended beyond the breast and nearby lymph nodes, metastasizing to various regions in the body. Common sites of metastasis include the bones, liver, and lungs, with the possibility of spreading to other organs or even the brain.

For patients diagnosed with Stage IV breast cancer, the primary approach to treatment involves systemic drug therapies. These therapies encompass hormone therapy, chemotherapy, targeted drugs, immunotherapy, or a combination of these modalities. In specific circumstances, surgical procedures and/or radiation therapy might also prove beneficial.

These treatments are designed to reduce tumor size or impede their growth while enhancing symptom management.

TRIPLE-NEGATIVE BREAST CANCER

Triple-negative breast cancer (TNBC) lacks estrogen and progesterone receptors, and it produces insufficient or negligible amounts of the HER2 protein. Consequently, hormone therapy and HER2-targeted drugs are ineffective in treating this form of cancer. Therefore, the primary systemic treatment option for TNBC is chemotherapy. Although TNBC typically exhibits an initial favorable response to chemotherapy, it also displays a higher tendency for recurrence compared to other types of breast cancers.

Triple-negative breast cancer stages I-III

In cases of early-stage triple-negative breast cancer (TNBC), the initial treatment approach is generally surgical removal of the tumor if it is small enough. This can involve breast-conserving surgery or mastectomy, along with a lymph node evaluation. Depending on specific factors such as tumor size and lymph node involvement, radiation therapy may be administered after surgery. Additionally, after surgical removal, adjuvant chemotherapy may be prescribed to reduce the risk of cancer recurrence.

For women with a BRCA mutation and specific tumor characteristics (tumor size between 2cm and 5cm or 1in and 2in, affecting underarm lymph nodes), a targeted drug may be recommended following adjuvant chemotherapy. This treatment has shown good results.

In some cases, chemotherapy is administered before surgery. If cancer is still found in the surgically removed tissue despite neoadjuvant chemotherapy, the doctor may propose further treatment options:

A targeted drug for some cases of BRCA mutation can be recommended, as it has been shown to reduce the risk of cancer recurrence and improve survival for some women.

These treatments aim to enhance patient outcomes and minimize the chances of TNBC returning.

Triple-negative breast cancer at stage IV

In cases where cancer has metastasized to other areas of the body (stage IV), chemotherapy is often the initial treatment.

For individuals with triple-negative breast cancer (TNBC) who possess a BRCA mutation and whose cancer has become resistant to standard breast cancer chemotherapy, alternative platinum-based chemotherapy drugs, as well as targeted drugs known as PARP inhibitors may be considered.

For advanced TNBC cases where the cancer cells express the PD-L1 protein, the primary treatment approach could involve a combination of immunotherapy and chemotherapy.

Approximately one in every five TNBC cases exhibits the PD-L1 protein.

When at least two other drug treatments have been attempted for advanced TNBC, another option to explore is an antibody-drug.

In cases of advanced triple-negative breast cancer (TNBC) with high levels of gene alterations known as microsatellite instability (MSI) or changes in mismatch repair (MMR) genes (MLH1, MSH2, MSH6, and PMS2), immunotherapy may be used. High TMB (tumor mutational burden) can make abnormal cells more likely to be identified and attacked by the immune system. Surgery and radiation are also potential treatments in certain situations.

TREATMENT OF BREAST CANCER INFLAMMATION

Inflammatory breast cancer (IBC) is a rare form of invasive breast cancer. It is characterized by the breast skin appearing red, feeling warm, and having a thick, pitted appearance similar to an orange peel. These changes are caused by cancer cells obstructing lymph vessels in the skin.

When diagnosed, inflammatory breast cancer is typically considered at least a stage III breast cancer because it has affected the lymph vessels and altered the skin. If it has spread to other parts of the body, it is classified as stage IV. These cancers grow rapidly and can be difficult to treat.

Regardless of the cancer's stage, participating in a clinical trial for new IBC treatments is a viable option. This is because IBC is rare, has a poor prognosis, and these trials often provide access to drugs not available in standard treatment

Treatment for stage III IBC

IBC in stage III refers to breast cancer that has not spread beyond the breast or nearby lymph nodes. The standard treatment approach usually begins with chemotherapy (chemo) aimed at reducing the tumor size. In cases where the cancer is HER2-positive, targeted therapy is administered in conjunction with chemo. After this, surgery, including mastectomy and lymph node dissection, is typically performed to remove the cancer. Radiation therapy often follows the surgical procedure. In some instances, additional chemo may be given after surgery but before radiation. If the cancer is hormone receptor-positive, hormone therapy is also provided, typically after completing all rounds of chemotherapy. The combination of these treatments has significantly improved survival rates over the years.

Surgery and additional therapies

If chemotherapy proves effective against the cancer, the next step is typically surgery. The standard procedure is a modified radical mastectomy, which involves removing the entire breast and the lymph nodes under the arm. Due to the extensive involvement of the breast and skin in Inflammatory Breast Cancer (IBC), breast-conserving surgeries like partial mastectomy or lumpectomy, as well as skin-sparing mastectomy, are not viable options. The reliability of sentinel lymph node biopsy (where only one or a few nodes are removed) in IBC is uncertain, so it is not considered an option either.

If the cancer does not respond to chemotherapy and the breast remains swollen and red, surgery cannot be performed at that stage. In such cases, other chemotherapy drugs may be attempted, or radiation treatment might be considered for the breast. If the cancer responds to this further treatment and the breast shrinks, making it no longer red, then surgery becomes a potential option.

Whether or not breast radiation is administered before surgery, it is given afterward, even if no cancer is believed to remain. This is known as adjuvant radiation, which helps reduce the risk of cancer recurrence. Typically, radiation is given five days a week for six weeks, but in some cases, a more intense treatment schedule (twice a day) may be used instead. The timing of radiation might be delayed until further chemotherapy and/or targeted therapy (like trastuzumab) have been given, depending on the amount of tumor found in the breast after surgery. If breast reconstruction is planned, it is generally postponed until after the radiation therapy, which often follows the surgery.

Treating stage IV breast cancer inflammation

Patients diagnosed with metastatic (stage IV) inflammatory breast cancer (IBC) undergo systemic therapy, which involves various types of treatment:

- Chemotherapy
- Hormonal therapy (for hormone receptor-positive cancer)
- Targeted therapy using HER2-targeting drugs (for HER2-positive cancer)
- Immunotherapy (if the cancer produces a protein called PD-L1)
- Targeted drug therapy using a PARP inhibitor, in cases where the woman has a BRCA mutation.

One or more of these treatments may be used, and sometimes, a targeted drug is combined with chemotherapy or hormonal therapy. In certain situations, surgery and radiation might also be considered as treatment options.

Considerations Regarding Breast Reconstruction

Many women may choose to undergo breast reconstruction surgery as a solution following breast cancer treatment. However, this option might not be suitable for everyone. It's essential to be aware of the potential risks and benefits associated with breast reconstruction and explore alternative treatment options.

Before deciding to remove a tumor or undergo breast surgery, it's crucial to have discussions with both your primary surgeon and a plastic surgeon specializing in breast reconstruction. By doing so, the surgical team can plan the most appropriate treatment course, even if you decide to delay reconstructive surgery.

The decision to opt for breast reconstruction can be influenced by various factors, including improving the fit of garments, permanently restoring breast shape, eliminating the need for an external breast prosthesis, and enhancing body image.

Although scars are a common outcome of breast reconstruction, they tend to fade with time, thanks to modern techniques that have minimized scarring. When wearing a bra, the reconstructed breasts should be sufficiently similar in size and shape to boost confidence when wearing different types of clothing.

Breast reconstruction can be beneficial after a lumpectomy or mastectomy, as it can improve appearance and restore self-confidence. However, it's crucial to understand that the reconstructed breast will not be an exact replica of the natural breast. If tissue from other body areas is used for reconstruction, such as the abdomen, back, thighs, or buttocks, these areas will also appear different after surgery. It's essential to discuss concerns about scars and changes in shape or contour with the surgeon, including their location, appearance, and sensation after recovery.

Risks associated with breast reconstruction.

Breast reconstruction surgery has potential risks and adverse effects that should be taken into consideration. Studies indicate that reconstruction does not cause breast cancer to return, and if cancer does recur, reconstructed breasts do not interfere with locating or treating the disease.

If you are considering breast reconstruction using an implant or tissue flap, it's essential to know that reconstruction rarely conceals the recurrence of breast cancer. However, this shouldn't be seen as a significant danger if you decide to undergo breast reconstruction. Some key points to consider are:

- You have the choice of undergoing breast reconstruction at the same time as your breast cancer surgery (immediate reconstruction) or at a later time (delayed reconstruction).
- If you prefer not to decide on reconstruction during breast cancer treatment, you can defer the decision until after surgery.
- Be mindful of avoiding unnecessary surgeries.
- Understand that not all reconstructive surgeries yield desired results, so communicate your expectations with your plastic surgeon.
- Scarring will occur on the breast and donor sites where tissue was taken (buttocks, abdomen, thighs, back).
- Reconstructed breasts may not feel the same as natural breasts and could have reduced sensitivity.
- Some individuals may have concerns with bleeding or scarring tendencies.
- Insufficient blood flow can lead to tissue death (necrosis) after reconstructive surgery, requiring additional procedures for correction.

- Previous surgeries, chemotherapy, radiation therapy, smoking, diabetes, obesity, and other factors can impact recovery.
- Surgeons may recommend delaying reconstruction, especially if you smoke or have health issues. Smoking cessation is advised at least two months before surgery for optimal healing. Some conditions may make reconstruction impossible.
- The surgeon may suggest reshaping the opposite breast to match the reconstructed breast (symmetrizing).
- Immediate reconstruction options may be limited if radiation is part of the treatment plan, as certain types of reconstruction performed before radiation can cause complications and affect the final appearance and feel of the reconstructed breast.
- Consult with a plastic surgeon before surgery to better understand your reconstruction options and set realistic expectations for the results.

Recognizing the significance of accessing guidance and support while navigating your reconstruction choices and adapting to the changes that may come with it is crucial. An intelligent starting point is to have conversations with your physician or other healthcare professionals. An excellent resource for assistance is the Reach to Recovery Volunteers, who are breast cancer survivors specially trained to aid others facing breast cancer or contemplating breast reconstruction. They can offer helpful recommendations, reading materials, and valuable advice. To find a local volunteer or program, you can request a referral from your cancer care team or get in touch with a support group at 1-800-4-CANCER (1-800-422-2345).

Alternative Breast Reconstruction Methods

Some women with breast cancer opt not to have breast reconstruction after surgery. They might choose this because they don't want additional surgeries or wish to resume normal activities quickly. Others are content with their appearance after cancer removal surgery. Cost can also be a factor, especially for women without health insurance. If they change their minds later, reconstruction is still possible but may be easier if decided before cancer surgery.

Some women may find breast reconstruction difficult or impossible due to other health conditions, such as obesity or issues with blood circulation caused by smoking or poorly controlled diabetes.

For those who don't want breast reconstruction, they have two options: using a breast form (a prosthesis worn inside the bra or attached to the body) to mimic the look and feel of natural breasts or choosing to go flat (not using a breast form).

Breast forms are designed to imitate the movement, texture, and weight of natural breast tissue. They help maintain a balanced posture and keep the bra in place. While they might feel awkward at first, they should become more comfortable with time. Once healed, a permanent breast form or prosthesis can be fitted.

Selecting the right bra is important when using a breast form. The bra you usually wear may work well or need slight modifications. For comfort during the healing process, bra extenders can be used to increase width. Women with larger breasts can relieve shoulder strap pressure with bra shoulder supports.

If you prefer wearing your breast form in a bra compartment, your regular bra can be adjusted, or you can find mastectomy bras with built-in compartments. If the breast form causes skin irritation, pocketed bras are recommended. Consult your doctor before wearing underwire bras.

For nighttime or more comfortable options, soft bras (leisure or night bras) are available at department stores, suitable for wearing breast prostheses under pajamas.

Options for Breast Reconstruction

There are numerous varieties of breast reconstruction techniques. Some are performed concurrently with mastectomy or lumpectomy, while others are performed later. Explore your available options.

Women who have undergone surgery to manage breast cancer have options for breast reconstruction. When determining the optimal type for you, you and your physicians should consider your health and personal preferences. Before deciding, take the time to research the available options and contemplate speaking with others who have undergone the same procedure.

Procedures for breast reconstruction

There are numerous types of reconstructive surgery, and the procedure frequently involves multiple operations. Allow yourself ample time to make the best decision possible. You should only decide on breast reconstruction after receiving complete information.

Implant reconstruction and tissue (flap) reconstruction are the two primary forms of breast reconstruction. Occasionally, both the implant and flap procedures are used to reconstruct a breast.

For all forms of breast reconstruction, future "touch-up" procedures, such as fat grafting and scar revisions, are frequently possible. Additionally, breast reconstruction can recreate the nipple-areolar region through a minor surgical procedure, tattooing, or a combination of the two. This is done to help the reconstructed breast resemble the original breast more closely.

Choosing the appropriate type of breast reconstruction

If you've chosen to have breast reconstruction, there are several factors to consider as you and your doctors discuss the best approach. Here are the important points to think about:

- The size and location of your breast cancer.

- Your breast size and shape.
- The extent of your breast cancer surgery, whether it's a lumpectomy or mastectomy, and whether you can keep your nipple.
- Whether you'll need additional cancer treatments apart from surgery.
- The amount of available tissue for reconstruction - some women may not have enough tissue, especially if they are very thin or have had a previous "tummy tuck."
- Decide if you want reconstruction for one or both breasts and if you prefer using your own tissue or donor tissue.
- Consider your insurance coverage and costs for the unaffected breast.
- Think about how quickly you want to recover from surgery.
- Be prepared for the possibility of multiple surgeries during the reconstruction process.
- Understand how different types of reconstructive surgery might affect other parts of your body.

Your surgeon will carefully assess your medical history and overall health to recommend the most suitable reconstructive options. They'll take into account your age, health, body type, lifestyle, and other factors. Don't hesitate to openly discuss your preferences, concerns, and priorities with your surgeon. It's essential to find a surgeon you feel comfortable with and to express any questions you have about the reconstruction. Your surgeon should explain the pros, cons, and risks associated with each treatment option.

- Questions for your surgeon.

Here are some initial questions to help you begin your decision-making process. Feel free to add more queries as they come to mind. The answers to these questions can guide you in making your choices.

- Am I eligible for breast reconstruction?
- When can reconstruction start?
- What are the advantages and disadvantages of immediate reconstruction (during cancer surgery) versus delayed reconstruction?
- Does reconstruction conflict with chemotherapy or radiation therapy?
- What are the available forms of reconstruction?
- What are the pros and cons of each option?
- Which reconstruction method do you recommend for me and why?
- What are the average costs for each type of reconstruction, and does my insurance cover them?
- How long will the recovery be for each type of reconstruction?
- How experienced are you in performing these procedures annually, and what results can I expect?
- Will my reconstructed breast look similar to my other breast?
- Should I consider surgery on the other breast for a balanced appearance?

- Is nipple reconstruction possible, and how is it done?
- How will my breast(s) feel after reconstruction, and will I have any sensation?
- What potential complications should I be aware of?
- Will there be pain, scarring, or changes in the areas where tissue is removed if a tissue flap is used?
- If a tissue flap is used, will I also need an implant for better contouring?
- How long will a breast implant last if I choose one?
- What type of breast implant will be used—smooth or textured, saline, or silicone?
- Will I need additional imaging exams based on the implant type, and will my insurance cover them?
- What breast changes can I expect over time?
- Is there a possibility of requiring additional surgery in the future due to potential complications?
- How will aging affect the breast reconstruction?
- How can I identify a ruptured implant?
- Are there any new reconstruction options, including clinical trials, that I should be aware of?
- Can you provide examples of typical outcomes from previous patients?
- Would it be possible to speak with other women who have undergone the same procedure?
- Feel free to add any other questions you may have to ensure you have all the information you need to make an informed decision.

TIP

When visiting your surgeon get someone to accompany you and take notes in your journal for further consultations.

In preparation for surgery

Your breast surgeon and plastic surgeon will provide you with detailed instructions before your surgery. These instructions may cover the following aspects:

- Smoking Cessation: You may be advised to stop smoking to prepare for the surgery.
- Vitamins, Medications, and Supplements: You will receive guidance on which vitamins, medications, and herbal supplements to take or avoid leading up to the surgery.
- Pre-Surgery Diet: You'll be given instructions on what to eat and drink before the surgery.

After the surgery, you should arrange for someone to drive you home, and you might need their assistance for a few days or more.

Regarding the location of your operation:

Breast reconstruction often involves multiple procedures. The initial step involves creating a breast mound, which can be done simultaneously with the mastectomy or at a later time. Typically, this procedure takes place in a hospital setting.

Subsequent follow-up procedures, like filling expanders and creating the nipple and areola, usually occur in an outpatient facility. However, the decision on the location of these procedures depends on the extent of surgery required and your surgeon's preferences. Make sure to inquire about these details from your surgeon.

Anesthesia

The initial phase of reconstruction is nearly always performed under general anesthesia. This means you will be given medications to induce sleep and block sensation during surgery.

Local anesthesia may suffice for subsequent procedures. This means that only the targeted area will be anesthetized. A sedative may also be used to induce a relaxed but conscious state. You may experience some discomfort.

Possible breast reconstruction surgery hazards

Breast reconstruction surgery carries inherent risks, and some women may face specific challenges during the process. Your surgeon will discuss these hazards with you, so if you have any uncertainties, don't hesitate to ask questions.

When preparing for breast reconstruction, talk to your surgeon about what you can expect and how to be fully ready for the procedure. Understand how your body will look and feel after surgery, along with the benefits and risks of the chosen reconstruction method. Here are some questions to ask your surgeon about the surgery:

- How much discomfort should I expect after surgery?
- How long will I need to stay in the hospital?
- Will I require blood transfusions?
- What is the expected duration of my recovery?
- How do I care for my surgical scars at home?
- Will I have a drain after surgery, and how should I care for it?
- Will I be given postoperative exercises, and when can I start them?
- What level of physical activity is safe at home?
- How do I handle arm swelling?
- When can I return to regular activities like work and driving?

It's essential to understand that the reconstructed breast may not exactly match your natural breast. However, breast reconstruction can improve your appearance and boost your self-confidence. If tissues from other parts of your body are used, those areas will also change after surgery. Discuss surgical scars and changes in shape with your surgeon to know what to expect.

Make sure your surgeon or other medical staff clarify the following aspects of your surgery:

- The type of anesthesia used during surgery and how pain will be managed.
- The location and duration of the surgery.
- Both short-term and long-term potential complications of the surgery.
- What to expect during the recovery period.
- The follow-up plan after surgery.
- The costs associated with the surgery.

After treatment

After breast reconstruction surgery, most women can return to their regular activities within six to eight weeks. If implants are used without flaps, the recovery time may be shorter. However, there are some important points to keep in mind:

- Different forms of breast reconstruction may not fully restore normal breast sensation, but some types could improve sensation over time.
- It may take around eight weeks for bruising and swelling to go down, so patience is necessary during the healing process.

- Complete tissue recovery and scar fading may take up to two years, but scars may never completely disappear.

- Consult with your surgeon about when you can wear conventional bras, as the type of surgery you had may influence the recommendation. After healing, underwires and lace in bras might be uncomfortable if they rub or press on scars.

- Follow your surgeon's guidance on when to start stretching exercises and normal activities, as this varies depending on the type of reconstruction. For about four to six weeks after reconstruction, avoid heavy lifting, strenuous sports, and certain sexual activities. Your surgeon will provide specific instructions.

- Some women may experience an adjustment period after breast reconstruction, similar to the time it takes to adjust to the loss of a breast. Talking with other women who have undergone breast reconstruction or seeking support from a mental health professional can be beneficial in managing anxiety and emotions.

- Silicone gel implants may rupture or seep without causing symptoms. Surgeons usually recommend periodic MRI scans for implants to check for any issues. Saline implants do not typically require this. Check with your physician about long-term follow-up and insurance coverage.

- If you notice any concerning symptoms like skin changes, swelling, lumps, pain, or fluid seeping from the breast, armpit, or flap donor site, contact your doctor immediately.

Women who have had a mastectomy for breast cancer usually do not need routine screening mammograms on the affected side due to insufficient tissue. However, they should still have mammograms on the other breast. If a suspicious area is found during a physical examination, a diagnostic mammogram, ultrasound, or MRI may be performed.

Always consult your doctor if you are unsure about the type of mastectomy you had or if you need mammograms.

Care Following Breast Cancer Treatment

After breast cancer treatment, many women experience relief but also fear the possibility of the disease returning and feel disoriented without regular contact with their cancer care team. Some women with advanced breast cancer may never fully eliminate the disease, leading to ongoing treatment to control and manage symptoms. Dealing with advanced, incurable breast cancer can be stressful and uncertain.

Even after completing treatment, it is essential to attend follow-up appointments for close monitoring. During these visits, physicians will inquire about symptoms and conduct examinations. In some cases, additional lab and imaging investigations may be necessary to determine the cause of symptoms.

Cancer treatments often cause adverse effects, which can last for varying durations. Doctor visits offer an opportunity to discuss concerns and ask questions. If cancer-related concerns arise between appointments, it's crucial to contact the doctor's office immediately.

Follow-up schedules are standardized but can vary based on factors like cancer type, stage at diagnosis, and current treatment. Initial follow-up visits may occur every few months after treatment completion, and their frequency may decrease over time, typically becoming annual after five years.

For women who have had breast-conserving surgery, mammograms are recommended 6 to 12 months after surgery and radiation, then annually. Those who had a mastectomy usually don't require mammograms unless one breast remains, in which case annual mammograms are necessary.

Women taking hormone drugs and having a uterus should undergo annual pelvic exams due to increased uterine cancer risk. Bone density screenings may be recommended for those taking aromatase inhibitors or undergoing menopause.

Blood tests and imaging tests are generally not part of standard follow-up, but they may be performed if symptoms or physical exams suggest cancer recurrence. In case of recurrence, additional tests, like CTCs and tumor marker level assessments, may be conducted to monitor treatment effectiveness.

Requesting a survivorship care plan from your physician is advisable. This plan may include a follow-up schedule, a summary of diagnosis and treatment, future testing recommendations, information on potential side effects, and lifestyle modification advice.

Breast cancer recurrence

If cancer comes back, the available treatment options will be determined based on where the recurrence occurs, past treatments, and your current health and preferences.

Women who have experienced breast cancer are still susceptible to other types of cancer, making it crucial to follow the American Cancer Society's recommendations for early detection of cancers, including colorectal and cervical cancer.

Women with a breast cancer history face a higher risk of developing other types of cancer.

For those who have had or currently have breast cancer, understanding ways to minimize the risk of cancer growth or recurrence, beyond standard treatment, becomes important. Activities like staying physically active, following a specific diet, or taking nutritional supplements have shown promise in breast cancer research.

Following breast cancer treatment, maintaining excellent overall health becomes even more crucial. Sustaining a healthy weight, engaging in regular physical activity, and adopting a balanced diet can not only reduce the risk of breast cancer recurrence but also protect against other health conditions.

Achieving a healthy weight

If you have had breast cancer, achieving and maintaining a healthy weight could reduce your risk. Numerous studies indicate that being overweight or obese (very overweight) increases the risk of breast cancer recurrence. It has also been associated with an increased risk of developing lymphedema, the result of damage or obstruction in the lymph system. This leads to the accumulation of fluid in soft tissues, causing swelling. It is a frequent issue often linked to cancer and its treatment. While it typically impacts an arm or leg, it can also affect other body areas.

Eating a nutritious diet

The majority of research on potential links between diet and the risk of breast cancer recurrence has focused on broad dietary patterns as opposed to particular foods.

Breast cancer survivors who consume more vegetables, fruits, whole cereals, chicken, and fish tend to live longer than those who consume more refined sugars, fats, red meats (including beef, pork, and lamb), and processed meats. (such as bacon, sausage, luncheon meats, and hot dogs).

Two large studies (WINS and WHEL) have examined the effects of reducing lipid intake after an early-stage breast cancer diagnosis. Women on a low-fat diet had a small reduction in the risk of cancer recurrence, according to one study. However, these women also lost weight as a consequence of their diet, which may have affected the results. The other study did not uncover a correlation between a low-fat diet and the risk of cancer recurrence.

After a diagnosis of breast cancer, many women have concerns about the safety of consuming soy products. Soybean products are an abundant source of isoflavones, which have estrogen-like effects on the body. Some studies have suggested that soy consumption may reduce the risk of breast cancer recurrence.

Alcohol

Even weekly consumption of a few alcoholic beverages increases a woman's risk of developing breast cancer. However, it is unclear whether alcohol influences the risk of breast cancer recurrence. Alcohol consumption can increase estrogen levels in the body, which could theoretically increase the risk of breast cancer recurrence.

It is advisable not to consume alcohol. Women who consume alcohol should limit themselves to no more than one drink per day to reduce their risk of developing certain types of cancer.

Having a good self-image both throughout and after breast cancer treatment.

In addition to the emotional, mental, and financial strains that cancer and its treatment can cause, many women with breast cancer must also deal with physical changes brought on by their treatment.

Some changes, like hair loss, may be temporary. However, even temporary changes can have a significant impact on how a woman views herself. Various options, including wigs, hats, scarves, and other accessories, are available to help women cope with hair loss. Alternately, some choose to identify themselves as breast cancer survivors through their baldness.

Other changes can be permanent, such as the loss of one or both breasts after surgery. Some women elect to undergo breast reconstruction surgery, while others choose not to. If you choose not to undergo breast reconstruction, you have the option of wearing a prosthesis.

Relationships after breast cancer

You may have sexual concerns after breast cancer. Some women may feel uncomfortable with their bodies due to physical changes, especially after breast surgery. There may be a loss of sensation in the affected breast. Other treatments for breast cancer, such as chemotherapy and hormone therapy, can change your hormone levels and may affect your sexual interest and/or response.

Relationship issues are also important. Your partner might worry about how to express love physically and emotionally after treatment, especially after surgery. But breast cancer can be a growth experience for couples – especially when both partners take part in decision-making and go to treatments.

Finding help and support after breast cancer treatment.

Regardless of the changes you may experience, it's important to know that there is advice and support out there to help you cope. Speaking with your doctor or other members of your healthcare team is often a good starting point to find it. There are also many support groups available, such as the American Cancer Society Reach To Recovery program. This program matches you with a local volunteer who has had breast cancer. Your Reach To Recovery volunteer can answer many of your questions and can give you suggestions, additional reading material, and advice. Remember that she's been there and will probably understand.

Some studies suggest that younger women tend to have more problems adjusting to the stresses of breast cancer and its treatment. It can feel socially isolating. Younger women might also be more affected by issues of sexuality or fertility (the ability to have children). Some younger women might be thinking about starting a family or having more children, and they might worry about how the cancer and its treatment might affect this. Others might have already started families and might worry about how family members might be affected. At the end of the book, I have listed some support groups that can help you with all your questions.

SUMMARY

Breast cancer affects both breasts in women and men. Not all tumors are cancer. Some are benign tumors like changes in fibrocystic tissue. Also, fibroadenomas and Papilomas.

There are two main types of breast cancer: Ductal Carcinoma In situ (DCIS) and Invasive Ductal Carcinoma. There are several ways of diagnosing breast cancer. Image is important in the detection of tumors. They are detected by mammograms that can be 2D or 3D. Other methods are ultrasound and Magnetic Resonance Imaging (MRI), Elastography, Optical Imaging, and Electrical Impedance Tomography.

Most breast cancers are treated with surgery and radiation. For more advanced stages, Chemotherapy is added along with other procedures when needed, such as Brachytherapy, Targeted Therapy, Immunotherapy, and Hormonal Therapy. Breast reconstruction is an option when a full mastectomy is performed. To prevent a recurrence, which could happen, achieving a healthy weight and exercise are highly recommended.

CHAPTER SIX

"Let food be thy medicine and medicine be thy food. "

— **Hippocrates**

FIFTH STEP

RECUPERATION AND NUTRITION

During treatment, it is very important to maintain a healthy diet. This will help your immune system to be in optimal condition. This is important because your body does not need additional issues that could compromise your immune system while it is doing its best at fighting cancer. You should try to keep eating as regularly as you did before the treatment started. I say, try because during treatments this will become more difficult as nausea and fatigue creep in. Regular schedules will become difficult to keep, and sometimes mouth sores will prevent you from consuming a solid diet. Be patient. These symptoms will pass.

I do not recommend you change your diet or your schedule at this point. Eat what you are used to, with just a few caveats. Stay away from sugar, tobacco, and alcohol. The changes that I recommend in this book in your daily diet are to be done after treatments, as they will be easier to do, and you will have additional energy to discipline yourself in doing so.

There has been a lot of talk about taking supplements and vitamins during treatment. I am not against this practice. You should talk to your doctor about this if you are so inclined. There have been several studies that recommend the taking of vitamins C and K during chemo and radiation, but most oncologists are against this practice. The reason is simple. Because of the complexity of drugs that go into chemotherapy, and the different reactions in people, your doctor will prefer to maintain the treatment following the protocol, and analyzing its effects, instead of introducing another variable into the equation, affecting the results of the treatment. Unfortunately, few oncologists have studied nutrition, because of the hardships of their specialty. For that reason, they do not include supplements and vitamins in their strategies to fight cancer during treatment.

Nutrition is then something to reckon with when we are in recuperation. A conscientious and healthy diet will help you recuperate your energy levels and have a positive mindset to get your life going again.

Detoxing after treatment.

This is an important step in your recuperation plans. The body has just been invaded by radioactive particles and combinations of drugs that will affect your system for some time.

The moment to detox your system is when you have stopped radiation and chemotherapy. There will be some medicines that you will still take, especially after surgery, yet the process must start as soon as possible. First thing, talk to your doctor and let him know what you intend to do. You do not want to start a new program that may affect post-surgery treatments, like antibiotics for infections. Notwithstanding, as soon as I went home, I started my program.

As my chemotherapy blew my taste buds away, and most of the food that I ate tasted bland, I could change habits and foods easily. To me, in the beginning, for example, broccoli tasted the same as French fries, so I just switched to broccoli. Yes, the consistency of the food was not the same, but that was a small price to pay. After a while, when I got my taste back, the broccoli was quite good!

The organs that are most affected by chemo and radiation are the skin, liver, digestive track, kidneys, mouth, hair follicles, and the sexual organs. The lymphatic system is as well. Depending on where the radiation is applied, it can also affect, the heart, lungs, brain, etc. So, as you can see, cancer treatments affect most organs and systems in the body. So, it is highly important to get all these organs cleaned and detoxified.

A detoxification function is then the purifying of all the organs and systems, by purifying the blood and the liver. The liver is important because this is where all the toxins are processed for elimination. Also, the body eliminates toxins through the kidneys, intestines, lungs, lymphatic system, and skin. So, when these organs and systems are compromised, they cannot function properly and they do not filter impurities, creating problems for the whole body.

The detox programs will help the body in its cleansing process through:

- Resting some organs through fasting.
- Stimulating the liver to cleanse the body.
- The promotion of toxin elimination through intestines, kidneys, and skin.
- Feeding the body with good nutrients.
- Cleansing the blood and improving circulation.

The first thing to do is to eliminate any toxic ingredients that are entering your body. Including alcohol, sugar, coffee, tobacco, saturated fats, and milk products. Try to stay away from toxic chemicals in personal items like deodorants, toothpaste, household cleaners, and shampoos. Try to substitute them with natural ingredients and products. Get rid of stress, as it triggers the release of stress hormones into your body, like adrenaline.

In my case, I went to a seven-day detox program that was simple to follow and that helped me get healthy.

I promoted the following products in my diet:

- Many fresh fruits and vegetables
- Fresh fish or canned in water or olive oil
- Two servings per week of lean meat or skinless chicken
- Legumes, like kidney beans, and lentils.
- Organic eggs
- Extra virgin olive oil and unprocessed coconut oil.
- Nuts, unsalted almonds, walnuts, macadamias, and cashews

Every morning I would take half a lemon juice in warm water. This would activate my liver and help my body maintain a healthy PH.

As part of my detox program, I started exercising. This made it easy to sweat it out, even by just walking briskly. Sweat cleans the body of toxins. Another way is to use a sauna and sweat it out. Just make sure that you are constantly drinking plenty of clean water.

Exercise. This is very important. It gets the blood flowing, gets your heart pumping, and the body is correctly oxygenated and cleansed of toxins. The idea is to do a 30 to 45 minutes aerobic workout. Yet not everybody will do it, as surgery could have been a major factor in your cancer treatment. But this does not mean that you should not get up and start walking as soon as possible. You should aim at doing it daily until you can walk 30 minutes and start breaking into a sweat. It took me an entire month to achieve it. But I was determined to do it, and I am glad I did, as it became one of my post- cancer habits, that I do till today.

Eat as many raw foods as possible. I would make myself lots of juices throughout the day, including veggie juices.

I learned to meditate. This was difficult as my mind kept on thinking of things I should do or fears of things not working out. I could do 20 minutes in the morning, and another 20 minutes in the early evening. This I did through a guided meditation program that I downloaded from the Internet. If meditation is new to you, I highly recommend downloading a program that will guide you through the process.

Eat probiotics. These will help your intestines to grow "good" bacteria and kill "bad" ones. Nonfat natural yogurts are the best.

Then, the easiest, drink a lot of water. More than you think you need. Water helps the blood, the kidney, and the digestive system to clean up. You will also sweat a bit more, but that is just the thing you want to do.

When you finish you will feel refreshed, and you will want to do it again after a while.

A NOTE ON SUGAR CONSUMPTION

Researchers have proved that cancer cells have a 'sweet tooth', and that they readily consume glucose for energy and reproduction. Some studies have found that elevated blood sugar levels and diabetes were risk factors for developing several types of cancer. Yet other studies have claimed that there is no firm evidence that directly links sugar to increase cancer risk, yet there is an indirect link. There is some controversy about the direct link between eating sugar and cancer, or if eating sugar causes cancer cells to reproduce faster or not.

It is my point of view that glucose per se does not cause cancer. Glucose feeds all cells in the body, especially brain cells. It is the source of glucose and the way the body absorbs glucose, that promotes cancer. Refined sugars used in the food industry for enhancing the taste of products lead to more consumption of the product (cravings) hence, weight and fat gain.

For this reason, I constantly mention to my readers that they should avoid refined sugars. I am not against the consumption of natural fructose in fruits and vegetables. They contain fiber when the body takes longer to digest and turn the sugars into glucose. In this way, we can keep the balance of insulin/sugar in the body at optimal levels.

In my diet, I have eradicated refined sugars. I have kept my weight in check, lessening the recurrence of cancer in my life. Yet sugar is not the only factor as I have mentioned before. The causes of cancer are many, and at least I will try to manage the factors that are under my control. Sugar consumption is one of them.

A note on sugar substitutes. I must be honest about it. In the beginning, I consumed a substitute with my tea, thinking that I was avoiding the deadly sugar syndrome, yet after a time my digestion was affected. I reasoned that this was because of the surgery, and the fact that my stomach was now a tube in my upper abdomen, acting as an esophagus. What I then found out was that most sugar substitutes affect your gut flora, changing the balance of your bacterial homeostasis. The gut microbiota. I had constant diarrhea until I reversed to drinking my tea with a little natural brown sugar or honey instead of a sugar substitute.

THE SYNERGY OF FOOD

Another controversy that exists in the nutritional world is whether vitamins and minerals in pills are effective. The controversy lies in whether vitamins and minerals that are synthesized are absorbed as well by the body compared to vitamins and minerals in their natural form. An example is when we take a complex B vitamin from a bottle. Will the body readily absorb it and help our body? Or is it better to eat cold fish or cod liver oil, to fortify your Vitamin B deficiency? I am convinced that the natural way is the most beneficial. This is because the multiple ingredients in natural foods help each other be absorbed by the body and help each other make its potency more effective. This "helping" of the ingredients is called synergy. So, it is not enough that you take a multivitamin every day, and then stuff yourself with "junk food!" Vitamins and minerals are best taken from natural ingredients, and we shall look at this more carefully. Please do not misunderstand, sometimes high doses of vitamins are needed, but this should be done with the supervision of your health provider, as negative reactions to this are possible, especially with minerals.

NATURAL FOOD

It has always amazed me when I go to the supermarket and see in the juice section multiple containers of fruit juices declaring that they are "natural". Well, any child knows what an orange looks like, and it is not a carton container! It is just as simple to look at the label and see that it probably comes from a concentrate, and has sugar and preservatives added. This is not "natural".

So, what is a "processed" product as opposed to a "natural" one? The simple answer is any product that has gone into a process of production and has gone into a package with additional ingredients to make it tastier and last longer. Sometimes, the products have added ingredients like sugar, salt, color dyes, and other chemical ingredients that increase the taste in the consumer's palate.

Natural food has an expiration date, and it is much faster than processed food. This is nature's way, and if the product stays bacteria free for a long period, it has an added product to it. Experiment. Buy a piece of bread from an organic bakery, and place that piece of bread next to a piece of loaf bread from the supermarket. It would surprise you how long the loaf of bread takes to grow mold. The nutritionist jokes that the bread is so bad that not even the bacteria will touch it!

We have forgotten why we eat. In our times, we are more concerned with taste, price, availability, and quantity than nutritional value. That's why some processed food seems to taste better. These products are packed with ingredients that enhance the flavor of things, yet they are so processed that they have lost most of their nutritional value. So, we eat to satisfy hunger, and yet most of the food we take will do more harm than good.

It is incredible how little we know about nutrition. We are a highly intelligent society, but unfortunately, we have assumed that the food that is offered to the public through supermarkets is good. I am not against having a burger and French fries now and then, but when it becomes a daily staple, that's when the problem starts. We have now become a society plagued by chronic diseases, like cancer, diabetes, Alzheimer's, high blood pressure, and stroke.

Now we have an additional reason to understand nutrition. We have experienced cancer, or somebody close to us is experiencing cancer. We must start reversing some factors that cause cancer. As they say, "Control your destiny, or someone else will".

I do not believe in radical behavior, so I do not propose a dramatization of our way of eating. I believe people should make the change by conviction, by a decision that is achieved by understanding the factors that affect our way of eating. We have cancer and we should help our bodies to fight the disease and maintain it at bay.

UNDERSTANDING NUTRITION

The objective is for you to understand the fundamentals of nutrition so that you can apply them to your daily life. I will try to make it as simple as possible so that you can start with your chosen path of nutrition immediately.

All foods have nutrients. It is the process of digestion that breaks up all these nutrients into substances that the body can absorb through the digestive system.

Nutrients are divided into macronutrients and micronutrients. Macronutrients are those that are needed by the body in larger quantities. Their function is to provide the body with energy that is measured in calories. These are nutrients that are needed in small quantities and are needed by the body as building blocks.

MACRONUTRIENTS.

These are divided into carbohydrates, proteins, fats, and water.

CARBOHYDRATES.

Carbohydrates provide fuel for the central nervous system and energy for working muscles. They also prevent protein from being used as an energy source. Carbohydrates enable fat metabolism, or the burning of fat.

They are highly important for brain activity, and they are influencers of mood, memory, focusing, and decision-making. We call them carbohydrates because they are molecules composed of carbon, hydrogen, and oxygen, divided into Simple and Complex Carbohydrates. The difference is the rate the body absorbs them, simple carbs being the fastest.

Simple carbohydrates contain just one or two sugars. Carbohydrates with one sugar, like fructose (found in fruits) and galactose (found in milk products), are called monosaccharides. Carbs with two sugars, such as sucrose (table sugar), lactose (from dairy), and maltose (found in beer and some veggies), are called disaccharides. Simple carbs are also present in candy, soda, and syrups. However, these are made with refined sugars and have no minerals, fiber, or vitamins, and we name them "empty calories" just leading to weight gain.

Complex carbohydrates (polysaccharides) contain three or more sugars. We often refer these to as "starch foods" and include cereals, whole grain bread, beans, peas, peanuts, potatoes, and corn.

It is then highly recommendable that you consume complex carbs instead of simple ones. Simple carbs are absorbed into the bloodstream faster and can spike your blood sugar.

In the body, carbs are broken down into smaller units of sugar, such as glucose or fructose. It is in the small intestine where these sugars are absorbed and then travel to the liver through the bloodstream. The liver then converts the sugars into glucose, which is then distributed to the whole body through the bloodstream, again accompanied by insulin produced by the pancreas, converting them into energy for basic body functions and physical activity.

The body can store up to 2000 calories in the liver and skeletal muscles as glycogen. Once glycogen stores are full, it is converted into fat. Glycogen deficiency causes the body to convert protein into energy, creating problems in the body. Proteins are an essential component to repair muscles.

Fiber is essential for food digestion. It feeds microbiota and promotes bowel movement, decreasing the risk of diseases such as coronary heart disease and diabetes.

PROTEINS.

These are macronutrients that support the growth and maintenance of body tissues. Amino Acids are basic building blocks of proteins, and we divided them into essential and nonessential. We get essential amino acids in food, like meats, fish, and legumes. The body produces the nonessential. Amino acids are probably the most abundant ingredient in the body after water, hence their importance. There are eight types of proteins in the body.

Hormonal. These are protein-based chemicals secreted by endocrine glands. Transported through the blood stream they function as messengers from cell to cell, each hormone affecting a certain type of cell, a target cell. These cells have receptors to which the hormones attach to transmit a specific signal. A good example is insulin, which is secreted by the pancreas and regulates levels of blood sugar in the body.

Enzymatic. These proteins speed up the metabolic functions in the body. Examples of these are liver functions, stomach digestion, blood clotting, and converting glycogen into glucose. An example of the process is the digestive enzymes that break down foods into simpler forms so that the body can absorb them.

Structural. These include keratin, collagen, and elastin. Collagen forms the connective tissue of your muscles, bones, tendons, skin, and cartilage. Keratin is the main structural component of hair, nails, teeth, and skin. Elastin is the protein that allows many tissues in the body to resume their shape after stretching or contracting.

Defensive. Antibodies or immunoglobulin are a core part of the defense system in our bodies. They are present in the white cells in our blood that attack bacteria, viruses, fungi, and other harmful microorganisms.

Transport. These proteins carry essential materials to our cells. Examples of these are Hemoglobin which carries oxygen to body tissues from the lungs. Serum albumin carries fats in our bloodstream and Myoglobin absorbs oxygen from hemoglobin and takes it directly to the muscles.

Receptor. These are located outside the cells and control the substances that enter or leave the cells, including water and nutrients.

Contractile. These are the motor proteins regulating the strength and speed of heart and muscle contractions. These are actin and myosin.

Storage. These proteins store mineral ions in the body. Ferritin, for example, regulates the amount of iron in the body, an essential ingredient in the production of hemoglobin.

FATS.

Provide energy, absorb certain nutrients, and maintain your core body temperature.

Although carbs are the primary source of energy in our bodies, the body turns to fat as a backup source of energy when carbs are depleted. Fats have double the calories of carbs, and they are hard to get rid of once the body stores them. Limiting your intake is the best way to do this.

Some types of vitamins, as we shall see, rely on fat for absorption and storage. So, you cannot discard the intake of fat.

Another function of fat is fat stored in adipose tissue. This tissue insulates the body and helps sustain a normal core body temperature. Other stored fat surround vital organs and keep them protected from sudden movements and outside impacts.

Good fat versus bad fat is simple to understand. Good fats are fats that come from vegetable oils, nuts, avocados, and cold-water fish like salmon or tuna. Yes, olive oil is good. These are also called monounsaturated or polyunsaturated fats. These raise the "good cholesterol" or HDL. (High-density lipoprotein) in the blood and fights "bad cholesterol".

Bad fats, or saturated and trans fats, are the bad guys. These are animal fats found in dairy products. These fats are also added to processed foods, so be aware of what you buy in the supermarket. They raise the "bad cholesterol" LDL (Low-density lipoprotein), which is the primary cause of hardened arteries and high pressure.

It is important to mention that sometimes we use lipids as a synonym for fats, yet fats are a subgroup of lipids and are also called triglycerides. Lipids also encompass molecules such as fatty acids and cholesterol. So, if your doctor says you must lower your triglycerides, it means you must lower your fat intake.

WATER.

60% of body weight is water. That's a lot of water. We use water in all our cells, organs, and tissues to regulate body temperature and other functions. Yet the body loses water through breathing, perspiration, and digestion. It is important to rehydrate by drinking fluids and eating foods that contain water.

Water protects your tissues, spinal cord, and joints. Keeping your body hydrated helps it keep optimum levels of moisture and liquids in these sensitive areas, as well as in the blood. In our joints and spinal cord, water acts as a protecting film around them.

Water helps our body to excrete waste through perspiration, urination, and defecation. This is an important function while you are receiving chemo and radiation therapy, as it gets rid of harmful chemicals and waste faster.

Water aids digestion, starting with saliva, the basis of which is water. Enzymes that break down food need water to dissolve food, breaking it into nutrients that are more accessible to the body. Water also helps soluble fiber to dissolve benefiting bowel movement.

Dehydration happens when the body loses liquids through sweat in high heat, exercise, or gastrointestinal disease, vomiting, and diarrhea. By the time you feel thirsty, your body is already dehydrated. The thirst mechanism lags our actual level of hydration. In elderly people, this is more acute. They confuse thirst with hunger, so they are more prone to dehydration. By just losing 1% of water in your body, your mood, attention, memory, and motor coordination will be impaired. Blood becomes more concentrated, kidneys will retain water, making you urinate less, and your heartbeat will rise compensating for blood pressure. A feeling of fainting may appear as if when you stand up too quickly.

You may also feel feverish, as it hinders body temperature. Cells become shrunken, and brain mass shrinks.

When you are going through treatment, these symptoms will probably appear. Make sure they are not from dehydration. You can tell if you're dehydrated. If your urine is clear, then you are ok. Darker urine shows you are dehydrated. Drink more water. There is a controversy between drinking fluids is the same as drinking water. I believe, through personal experience, that drinking water is better because unfortunately coffee and tea have other ingredients that affect absorption. Sports drinks do not hydrate you. They probably give you some energy because of the content of glucose, but they help you dehydrate as their minerals and glucose need water to dissolve them. Alcohol does the same. A beer does not hydrate you. I am sorry.

MICRONUTRIENTS.

They are nutrients we need in fewer quantities, yet they are just as important for the body's metabolism, the immune system, the production of energy, and the maintenance of the muscular, nervous, and bone systems. Most of the nutrients come from outside sources. Vitamins and minerals compose the micronutrients.

VITAMINS

We need these nutrients for the metabolism of the body, and to keep in optimum condition our immune system. We divided vitamins into two groups. They are soluble in water or fat. The water-soluble vitamins travel freely in the body and the kidneys eliminate any excess of them, avoiding this way dangerous overdose and becoming toxic. Not so with the fat-soluble, which are stored in the body and pose a risk of toxicity when consumed in excess.

WATER-SOLUBLE VITAMINS

Vitamin B1

Also known as Thiamine, comes from the vitamin B complex family. It plays an important role in the correct functioning of the nervous system and healthy cardiovascular activity. It also plays an important part in the conversion of carbs into glucose and the breakdown of fats and proteins.

We can find vitamin B1 in the liver and yeast as a primary source. We can also find it in whole-grain cereals, pork, rye, and kidney beans. Other sources include potatoes, mushrooms, asparagus, tuna, spinach, green peas, eggplant, Brussels sprouts, spinach, and romaine lettuce.

Another health benefit is boosting energy production. It is an anti-aging substance, that stimulates digestion, prevents Alzheimer, enhances memory, improves appetite, and boosts the immune system.

Vitamin B2

Also known as Riboflavin plays a critical role in the production of energy by converting carbs into sugars, which then fuel the function of many parts of the body. Its antioxidant properties help the body stay young. We find vitamin B2 in dairy products, liver, lean meats, oysters, broccoli, mushrooms, salmon, avocado, eggs, asparagus, spinach figs, and many others.

Other health benefits include protecting the skin and hair and keeping them healthy. Promotes development and growth, increases blood flow, protects the digestive track, treats anemia, and helps to prevent cancer.

Vitamin B3

Also known as niacin, plays a crucial role in different functions in the body. It reduces the risk of heart disease, improves mental health, treats diabetes, alleviates symptoms of arthritis, lowers the levels of triglycerides, and treats impotence.

Luckily, this vital vitamin is easily available to the body through the ingestion of meats, eggs, turkey tuna, oats, brown rice, cheese, milk, legumes, fish, whole grains, nuts, and dried beans.

Vitamin B5

We also know this vitamin as Pantothenic Acid and it is important because of its specific functions. This vitamin stimulates hormonal production, relieves stress, keeps the heart healthy, and reduces fatigue. The nervous system and a healthy brain rely on it.

We find it in chicken liver, salmon, sundried tomatoes, avocados, corn, broccoli, mushrooms, yogurt, and cauliflower.

Vitamin B6

Also known as pyridoxine, that helps to keep the skin and nerves healthy, fight infection, keep blood sugar at normal levels, produce red blood cells, and get some enzymes working properly. We find this vitamin in cereals, beans, nuts, peas, meat, poultry fish, eggs, and bananas.

Vitamin B6 is being studied in the prevention of hand-foot syndrome (tingling in the hands and feet) caused by certain drugs in chemotherapy.

Vitamin B7

Also known as Vitamin H or Biotin. This vitamin helps mainly to maintain healthy hair and skin. It fights bacteria and boosts the metabolism in the body, which is important to lose weight. Biotin also helps to prevent cramps.

Other health benefits include the aid of metabolizing carbohydrates and proteins, controlling blood sugar, helping multiple sclerosis, and balancing cholesterol levels.

It is readily available in egg yolk, cheddar cheese, salmon, avocado, mushrooms, nuts, soybeans, cauliflower, leafy greens, bananas, and walnuts.

Vitamin B8

Also known as Inositol. It is an important part of normal cell functions in the body. It is effective in controlling hypertension, and depression, and improves cognitive functions.

We can find this vitamin in beef, cereals, citrus fruits, green leafy vegetables, soy, nuts, and in whole grains.

Vitamin B12

This vitamin is important in the manufacturing of red blood

cells, DNA, RNA, and tissues, maintaining nerve cells healthy.

We find it in the liver, meat, poultry, eggs, shellfish, and dairy products.

It is being studied together with folate, for the prevention of certain types of cancers.

Folic acid

Also called folate, is crucial in the manufacture of red blood cells, maintaining in an optimal condition, the heart, blood vessels, and the optimal fetus development of the brain and spinal cord.

We can find sources of this vital ingredient in whole-grain bread and cereals, green vegetables, orange juice, lentils, beans, and yeast. Folic acid is being studied together with vitamin B12 for the prevention and treatment of cancer.

Vitamin C

Also known as ascorbic acid, is the king of vitamins. Not only does it prevent and treat the common cold, scurvy, and hypertension, but it also heals cataracts, prevents cancer, promotes good mood, slows down aging, promotes a healthy cardiovascular system, and boosts the immune system.

We readily find it in tomato, red and green peppers, citrus fruits, broccoli, kiwis, strawberries, cabbage, potatoes, spinach, pineapple, and papaya as in many other fruits and vegetables.

I would particularly like to make a special mention of its properties to fight cancer. High doses of Vitamin C given intravenously have proven to kill cancer cells, especially in patients with pancreatic and lung cancer.

Vitamin C breaks down easily producing hydrogen peroxide that damages selectively cancer cell's DNA and tissue. Cancer cells with lower levels of catalase, a substance that can neutralize hydrogen peroxide, are likely to be more responsive to high doses of vitamin C therapy. Studies are going underway to determine what cancer cells are low in catalases.

FAT-SOLUBLE VITAMINS

Vitamin A.

Also known as retinol has many functions in the body. Besides helping the eyes adjust to the light, it plays an important role in bone growth, tooth development, cell division, reproduction, gene expression, and regulating the immune system. The skin, eyes, and mucous membranes in the mouth, nose, throat, and lungs depend on this vitamin to maintain moist. This is especially important during chemotherapy. Vitamin A is also a powerful antioxidant that can prevent certain cancers.

The best sources of this vitamin are dairy products, fish, and liver. Beta-carotene is an antioxidant that the body converts to vitamin A. It can be found in red and orange vegetables like carrots, pumpkins, winter squash, apricots, and green leafy greens.

Adequate vitamin A intake from plant foods has been linked to the reduction of certain types of cancers, including Hodgkin's lymphoma, as well as cervical, lung, and bladder cancers. It is important to underline that these studies used natural plant beta-carotene and not in pill form.

Vitamin A. Investigations, as a cancer aid, are inconclusive at this moment, although it is essential in its natural form for the correct cell division.

Vitamin D

It plays an important role in the body's use of calcium and phosphorous. It increases the amount of calcium that is absorbed by the small intestine to maintain bones and teeth.

We find Vitamin D in dairy products fortified with vitamin D, oily fish, including herring, salmon, trout, and sardines, as kin cod liver oil. Sunlight also produced vitamin

D in our skins. Unfortunately, UV light in the sun's rays can also affect the cell structure in our skin, causing skin cancer. It is important to take small doses of sunlight at its lower points on the horizon and to use skin protection.

Vitamin E

Also known as Tocopherol, is a powerful antioxidant protecting red blood cells, essential fatty acids, and vitamins A and C from being destroyed. Research has led to the suggestion that taking vitamin E can prevent cancer. The antioxidants have been proven to work better when taken from fruits and vegetables.

We can find vitamin E in almonds, peanuts, hazelnuts, vegetable oils, and green leafy vegetables, like spinach and broccoli.

Important studies have been made to support the link between selenium and vitamin E in the prevention of prostate cancer. The studies have also linked Vitamin E to the improvement of radiation therapy in cancer cells, without damaging normal cells.

Vitamin K

Vitamin K occurs naturally as a byproduct of good bacteria in the intestines, and it plays an essential role in normal blood clotting, bone health, and the metabolism of proteins for blood, bones, and kidneys.

Sources of vitamin K are kale, spinach, turnip greens, Brussels sprouts, broccoli, cauliflower, and cabbage, also fish, liver, meat, eggs, and cereals.

Vitamin K2 (menaquinone) has been shown to suppress the growth and invasion of human *hepatocellular carcinoma*, a common and deadly liver cancer.

Vitamin K reduces solid cancer tumors in vitro and animal studies, which can lead to the improvement of cancer survival rates for liver and prostate cancers.

IMPORTANT NOTE.

Fat-soluble vitamins can be toxic when exceeding the recommended daily allowance, so be careful when ingesting vitamin supplements. Talk to your health provider.

MINERALS

Elements that are found on the earth. They act as the building blocks of our diet. Like vitamins, they play multiple roles in our bodies. Some minerals have structural functions like calcium and phosphorous, these minerals are the key components of bones and teeth. Yet Calcium has other critical functions. Along with other minerals like sodium, chlorine, potassium, and magnesium, calcium is a regulator of cell function. The minerals sodium, chloride, and potassium act as electrolytes, maintaining the balance of fluids inside and outside of cells; along with calcium, it controls the movement of nerve impulses.

Calcium

You have more calcium in your body than any other mineral. It handles various functions. The body stores over 99 percent of its calcium in the bones and teeth, helping in their formation and maintenance. The rest is spread around the body in the blood and muscles. Your body needs this mineral to help muscles and blood vessels contract. It is also important in the secretion of hormones and enzymes from different organs. Calcium plays an important role in the sending of messages through the nervous system.

Sources of calcium include dairy products, such as milk, cheese, yogurt, leafy green vegetables, fish with edible soft bones, like sardines, and salmon. We can also get calcium from calcium-enriched foods.

The exact amount of calcium you need varies depending on your age and other factors. Growing children and teenagers need more calcium than young adults. Older women need plenty of calcium to prevent osteoporosis, a disease that thins and weakens the bones and becomes brittle.

Calcium has been associated with lowering the risk of colorectal cancer.

Vitamin D and calcium are strongly correlated and share similar anticarcinogenic effects on mammary glands. "Vitamin D, Calcium, and **Breast cancer Risk: A Review**". Yan Cui, and Thomas E Rohan, published in August 2006 in National Library of Medicine. [viii]

Sodium

The body needs sodium for the functions of muscles and nerves. It keeps the right balance of fluids in your body.

The body needs sodium for the functions of muscles and nerves. It keeps the right balance of fluids in your body. The kidneys play an important role in this function, as they control sodium levels in the blood. The kidneys cannot get rid of excess sodium, leading to high blood pressure. In the US, people get more sodium in their diets than is needed. A key to healthy eating is choosing foods low in sodium and avoiding processed foods. The primary source of sodium in our diet is table salt. Other sources that you should look out for are yeast bread, cold cuts, savory snacks, cheese, bacon, frankfurters, sausage, ketchup, ready-to-eat cereal, French fries, cakes, and pies.

Patients with **lung** cancer can develop low levels of calcium, which can create symptoms such as nausea/vomiting, headaches, confusion, and even seizures. If you have these symptoms, advise your doctor.

Chloride

It is one of the major minerals in the body and helps fluid levels remain balanced by working closely with both sodium and potassium. Chloride works by maintaining fluid levels outside the cells in the body. It is an important contributor to the making of hydrochloric acid in the stomach, which is an important digestive fluid. Because it is an electrolyte, it plays a crucial role in the fluids throughout the body, including lymph, blood, and fluids found on the inside and surroundings of cells. The principal source is table salt. As with sodium, too much chloride can cause hypertension.

High doses of Sodium Chloride, or table salt, are linked to gastric cancer. Salted and pickled foods are the most dangerous. The findings of many epidemiological studies suggest that high dietary salt intake is a significant risk factor for gastric cancer and this association was strong in the presence of Helicobacter (H.) pylori infection with atrophic gastritis.

Potassium

An essential mineral found inside the cells of our bodies. It is an important nutrient for the proper function of all body cells tissues and organs. The specific roles of this mineral include nerve function, blood pressure regulation, and muscle control. It is also an electrolyte that conducts electricity. One of the important roles of potassium is its ability to relax blood vessels and excrete excess sodium, which both lowers blood pressure.

We can find potassium in vegetables, fruits, legumes, and meats. Bananas, oranges, cantaloupe, honeydew, apricots, prunes, raisins, and dates are high in potassium. Other sources include spinach, cooked broccoli, potatoes, mushrooms, cucumbers, zucchini, eggplant, and leafy green vegetables.

In an article published in the National Cancer Institute on March 28, 2019, scientists discovered that "dying cancer cells release the chemical potassium, which can reach high levels in some tumors. They reported that elevated potassium causes T cells to maintain a stem-cell-quality or 'stemness' that is closely tied to their ability to eliminate cancer during immunotherapy." [ix] The findings showed that potassium could enhance the fight against cancer during immunotherapy.

Phosphorous

Phosphorous is abundant in the body. This mineral is essential together with calcium, in the strength of the bones. Phosphorous plays an important role in helping body tissues grow, maintain health, and repair when needed. It plays an important role in the storage and production of energy. This mineral maintains a balance of pH in the body and helps kidneys maintain proper function.

Sources of this mineral include tuna, lean pork chops, tofu, low-fat milk, lean chicken breast, scallops, lentils, squash, pumpkin seeds, beef, and quinoa, among others.

Researchers linked high contents of phosphorus from processed food to alterations in cell functions that lead to damaging effects. Examples of possible adverse health effects include cancer, obesity, and hypertension.

Magnesium

This mineral maintains most of the body functions which regulate the vital processes of the heart for a healthy cardiovascular environment and bone density. It also drives the balance of our fuel source, as it is an important ingredient in the production of energy in the cells. This mineral protects our DNA and the synthesis of it. It regulates our electrolyte balance and is an active ingredient in over 300 enzymes in the body. Sources of magnesium include dark chocolate, avocados, nuts, legumes like lentils, beans, peas, soybeans, tofu, whole grains, fatty fish like salmon, mackerel, halibut, bananas, and leafy greens.

A study published in 2000 found that almost half the cancer patients admitted to the intensive care unit had low magnesium levels. It could be a side effect of treatment. Cisplatin, a chemotherapy drug used for various types of cancer, can cause several serious side effects, including magnesium deficiency in up to 90% of patients. The results of a 2008 study show that preventive magnesium supplementation can prevent side effects and decrease the severity of the drug's kidney damage without interfering with the anticancer effects of the drug. There was a longer survival rate.

TRACE MINERALS

These are minerals that are important in smaller quantities.

Iron

The mineral is essential to the body. It helps to keep oxygen circulating in the body and aids important chemicals to be transported in the bloodstream. We find iron is in every cell of the body, and is a primary component in hemoglobin, the protein that carries oxygen. Iron aids other body proteins that are essential for energy metabolism and respiration. This mineral is a part of the synthesis of DNA, and it contributes to proper immune function.

There are two forms of dietary iron: heme and non-heme. Heme iron comes from hemoglobin. We find it in animal foods that originally contained hemoglobin, like red meats, fish, and poultry. The body absolves the heme iron more than the non-heme iron derived from plants. Foods that are rich in this mineral include shellfish, spinach, liver and other organ meats, legumes, red meat, pumpkin seeds, quinoa, turkey, broccoli, tofu, and dark chocolate.

Iron deficiency is a common side effect of chemotherapy. This occurs with many of the drugs currently in use. Chemotherapy attacks all rapidly growing cells, not just cancer cells, like the cells in the bone marrow that are used to replace white blood cells, red blood cells, and platelets, are some that are affected. Doctors do blood counts before each chemotherapy infusion, and if the red blood cells are low, they will delay chemotherapy. Some patients are treated with medications that stimulate the production of blood cells so that chemotherapy can continue. Anemia can also be the first symptom of colon cancer. The most common symptoms of anemia are:

- Feeling weak or tired all the time.
- Shortness of breath.
- Increase susceptibility to infection.
- Cold hands and feet.

- Pallor.

Zinc

Has several roles in metabolism and immune functions and we need it to produce retinal or vitamin A. It has a major role in the growth and development of children, and it regulates behavior and affects taste. It is involved in cell reproduction, growth, and metabolism. It is highly important to the immune system.

Sources of this mineral include plain yogurt, ground meat, oysters, broccoli, lean sirloin steak, and crab.

Supplements of zinc can significantly inhibit the proliferation of esophageal cancer cells, according to studies. This mineral is important in cancer prevention.

Iodine

It is an essentially non-metallic mineral, necessary for normal thyroid function as it is a major component of the hormones T3 and T4. These two hormones are extremely important as they regulate the basal metabolism rate o and temperature. The basal metabolism rate is the rate of energy expenditure in vital cellular activity.

Human data, together with animal and in vitro models, all confirm the theory that iodine compounds are essential in the health and proper differentiation of tissues.

We find iodine in seafood. Shellfish, white fish, seaweed, and plants that grow in rich iodine soils. Cod fish is an excellent source of iodine, as are dairy products like yogurt, iodized salt, shrimp, tuna, eggs, prunes, and lima beans.

Selenium

This mineral plays an important part in the enzymatic function of the human body. There is a link to selenium aiding in the stimulation of antibody production following a vaccination. It aids male fertility and can act as an antioxidant. This is especially important as it works alongside other antioxidants, like vitamins C and E, in neutralizing free radicals in the body that are linked to the development of various cancers and heart diseases.

Sources of selenium are Brazil nuts, fish, ham, enriched foods, pork, beef, turkey, chicken, cottage cheese, eggs, brown rice, sunflower seeds, baked beans, mushrooms, oatmeal, spinach, milk, yogurt, lentils, and bananas.

Selenium is a powerful mineral. Your cell's defense against cancer depends on it. This mineral is a central compound of the enzymes that knock out free radicals, the unstable molecules that attack your cells and ultimately lead to cancer. It also plays a role in recycling antioxidants through the body. These antioxidants, such as vitamin E, then lower the risk of cancer by preventing free radicals from damaging cells. "How selenium helps Protect against Cancer" Healthline Sep.18, 2018. [x]

Copper

Its chief function is to act as a catalyzer for different biochemical reactions in the body, especially in the synthesis of hemoglobin. Another important role is in the production of collagen, elastin, melanin, and neurotransmitters. It is a natural defense against free radicals.

The best sources of copper are Oysters, raw kale, mushrooms, sesame seeds, cashew nuts, beans, prunes, avocados, goat cheese, and tofu.

Depriving malignant tumors of their copper supply may be a potent antiangiogenic strategy for stabilizing patients with advance cancer.

Manganese

We find this mineral in the bones, liver, pancreas, and kidneys. Manganese helps in the formation of connective tissue, bones, sex hormones, and blood clots. It plays a role in fat and carbohydrate metabolism, calcium absorption, and blood sugar regulation.

We can get it from mussels, toasted wheat germ, tofu, sweet potatoes, pine nuts, brown rice, lima beans, chicken peas, spinach, pineapple, oats, and rye.

Chromium

There is some evidence that this mineral interacts with thyroid functions. It plays an important role in the formation of DNA and RNA.

Chromium is present in mussels, Brazil nuts, Oysters, dried dates, pears, tomatoes, mushrooms, and broccoli.

Research teams from Australia have shown in early studies that taking nutritional supplements containing chromium over a long period can lead to the risk of cancer. Usually, people take this supplement to aid weight loss and type 2 diabetes.

Molybdenum

It is one of the essential ingredients in the metalloenzyme in the body that helps to convert purines into uric acid. Too much purine in the body causes gout. These enzymes also clean the body of sulfites and break down aldehydes, all toxic to the body.

Sources of this mineral are legumes, almonds, cashews, peanuts, cheese, yogurt, eggs, whole grains, and leafy green vegetables.

Studies have shown that low levels of Molybdenum seem to add to the risk of esophageal, and forestomach, cancer.

Fluoride

Fluoride works with other minerals to mineralize bones and teeth. Too much of this mineral can be detrimental to teeth.

Sources of fluoride include tap water, raisins, blue crab, shrimp, table wine, and grape juice.

There has been a lot of debate about the link between fluoride and osteosarcoma. There is no proof that this is true.

The information on quantities or quality of vitamins and minerals can be overwhelming. Having to choose the right vitamin or the right mineral is daunting. Especially when you read an overdose can have adverse results. So, what to do? A multivitamin is not the answer. What I highly recommend is to eat a balanced meal with as many natural vegetables, legumes, and fruits as possible. Organic products if they are available.

This will ensure you are getting the right vitamins and minerals you need, and you will let your body decide through homeostasis to bring the right balance to your body. Regarding meats for protein, I firmly believe that they are important, especially as they contain certain amino acids which are necessary for the body and are not found in vegetables, legumes, or fruits. Fish can be an important source of these amino acids, and you will save calories. If you need meat in your diet, I recommend a small portion of lean meat, but only twice a week for one meal. What is a small portion? The size of your palm would be good. Eggs are a significant source of vitamins and minerals, and I ate them twice a week.

To me, it became obvious. I started eating with my brain and not with my stomach. I decided in my head what I would eat, not letting my mouth dictate what I was going to consume. After a while, it becomes routine, and I started enjoying different ingredients, herbs, and spices to make them more interesting and enticing.

MINOR DIETARY ELEMENTS

Maintaining a healthy diet is quite easy. What is difficult is to change our habits of eating. I recommend the following points to follow:

- Avoid processed food. These foods are altered from their original state. Food processing can be as basic as freezing, canning, baking, and drying. The problem also arises from the fact that most of these foods have additional salt, sugar, or fats, added plus conservatives. Avoid tinned food, smoked and cold cuts, including sausages.

- Eat everything natural that you can, but the proportion of servings must change. It is customary to give preference to protein products, meats, poultry, fish, and dairy products. These are predominant, and we then have a side portion of vegetables. Change this proportion, raise vegetable intake, and minimize protein products.

- Eat less and more often. Eat five times a day and eat fewer amounts of food. This will help your organism. There will be meals with only vegetables or legumes. Eat protein only once a day, preferably fish.

- If you need protein, choose vegetable protein to supplement your diet.

- Use supplements with your diet not instead of your diet.

- Wash and disinfect your veggies and fruit, especially those that you do not peel.

FOOD, HERBS, AND SUPPLEMENTS TO FIGHT CANCER

There are multiple books on diets for cancer patients. I do not want to delve into diets.

This book gives you a comprehensive summary of all the knowledge I have accumulated. Guide you through the maze of information, avoiding all the fake and false promises that are offered online.

I do not believe in miraculous products that cure cancer. Cancer is a complex disease, and each cancer is different, as our DNA is different. Curing cancer is a complex process, and I believe that a combination of traditional medicine with alternative medicine is the best way to go about it. In my mind, a cancer patient should use all the weapons available in modern medicine, and then combine them with alternative medicine to help the body recover and prevent cancer cells from reproducing themselves uncontrollably again. To put it more plainly. I went through with the best treatment available at the time, radiation, chemotherapy, and surgery, which left me depleted, and then I started helping my body with good nutrition and scientifically proven supplements.

I must mention that there is a constant fight between big pharma and naturalists regarding the efficacy of certain products. Yet there are studies done in other countries that are accepted as official remedies for cancer. We can find these in China, Japan, and Europe, where doctors readily prescribe homeopathy ingredients. It is interesting to find that in

France, for example, you go to a pharmacy for a cold remedy, and the certified pharmacist will prescribe Paracetamol, Echinacea, with zinc and vitamin C. Nothing else.

Researchers are constantly disproving each other. Normally, the official statement from the government regarding natural treatments is that the studies are inconclusive. The way to go is to find out who sponsored the study, or what university or organization you trust did it. Make sure that the source of the information is trustworthy.

In all my research and studying, several products appear constantly in studies referring to cancer. These ingredients are accepted and sometimes proven to fight cancer. These products are the ones that I use in my daily life and have kept me free of cancer.

How do I know? After my first treatment in 2003, I went back to my old life and my old habits. The cancer appeared again in 2007. I have been free from cancer ever since, and I did it by cleaning up my act and following all the advice I am giving you here, hoping it will work for you.

Green Tea.

My first choice in a product to fight cancer is Green Tea. Its origin is China, *Camellia sinensis*, and there are several varieties of it, depending on the region of growth. The benefits this plant gives us are multiple because it concentrates several polyphenols called catechins. One of these, EGCG (epigallocatechin gallate), is a specially potent molecule that prevents the growth of cancer cells and the formation of blood vessels that feed tumors.

Multiple studies published by the National Center for Biotechnology in the National Library of Medicine showed that the antioxidants in green tea inhibit the cancerous cell from entering its "Cellular Cycle" forcing it to stop its growth. The EGCG stimulates the increase of other cellular proteins, which makes it difficult for cancer cells to develop. "Epigallocatechin Gallate (EGCG) Is the Most Effective Cancer Chemopreventive Polyphenol in Green Tea" [xi]

Also, in other studies, researchers showed EGCG promoted the death of cancerous cells in prostate cancer.

For tumors to keep on growing, they need nutrition, creating blood vessels to feed them and to distribute cancer cells to other tissues. This is called "angiogenesis". In other studies, they showed that the consumption of tea inhibits the growth of several tumor types in animals, including cancer of the **lung** and esophagus. They have associated the drinking of green tea with a lower incidence of human cancer.

Green tea is the product of the plant *Camellia sinensis.* The leaves of the plant are picked and dried. They do not undergo the withering and oxidation process that is used to make oolong teas and black teas. This aging process destroys many of the polyphenols, which are beneficial to our health.

There are many varieties of this tea. They depend on the plant and the region it grows. Conditions, horticulture methods, production processing, and time of harvest are also factors. It is important to mention that Japanese green tea, especially Sencha, Gyokuro, and Matcha, are some of the highest in the content of polyphenols, specifically EGCG.

Before I drank green tea, I was a coffee drinker. Green tea did not have any appeal to me. After my treatments and reading different studies, I tried it. The taste at the beginning was not very appealing to my palate. So, I started drinking green tea in combination with Jasmin. This was delicious, and now I drink it every morning as my first drink of the day. A hot mug of this combination during the sunrise is one of my happiest moments of the day. During the day, I now drink the Japanese version, called Sencha, which is higher in polyphenol content. If you are not used to it, try first the milder versions of Chinese teas, and then as time goes by, you will graduate to Japanese green teas.

Why not just take EGCG directly in a pill? It is my firm belief that the catechins in green tea do not work by themselves. Not one substance works towards our objective. I believe polyphenol works together with other substances that are present in the tea leaves. Here lies the difficulty of letting science dictate what is good or what is bad.

Green tea ingredients are extremely complex. It contains over 200 bioactive compounds, and their concentrations vary from region to region depending on the species. Can you imagine the cost and the effort that studies in vitro and in vivo would take to isolate each ingredient? Test them one by one, and then in combinations. Make tests to determine what compounds and at what concentrations and combinations to use. Then test them with different cancer cells. It would take a lifetime! All that work and cost for a study that cannot be patented as a product. Not likely. Somebody must pick up the tab, and it will not be a pharmaceutical company that cannot make money with this research.

This is the reason universities with special grants do these investigations. Thank God. They are an invaluable source of information. I am not against big pharma. Some companies are ethical and spend lots of money on research. That's their business. I thank them for all the drugs we take for specific illnesses, yet all their drugs are patented and costlier as we finally have to pay for all their effort. Cancer is a complex illness, and we should fight it with all the available means.

SPICES

Turmeric.

This spice is widely used in Asia, especially in India. Its principal ingredient is curcumin. The plant *Curcuma longa* comes from the ginger family, and its root is part of the plant that is used to make this yellow spice. This spice is another of the substances I highly recommend when starting your path to recovery. The powder has been used for centuries in Ayurveda medicine in India. Its properties include anti-inflammatory and antioxidant benefits. The anti-inflammatory property is one of the strongest in the botanical world, and it is used to stop chronic inflammation in the body. I would like to make a parenthesis here. We know that all toxic invasions to our bodies provoke an inflammatory reaction. This is a healthy reaction from our immune system. Notwithstanding, if the invasion becomes constant, then the inflammation also becomes constant, becoming what is called chronic inflammation. This inflammation can detonate a rapid cellular reproduction cycle, that after a time, becomes uncontrollable. Here is where cancer cells make their appearance. The inflammation process is natural in the body. We have all heard of dermatitis, colitis, conjunctivitis, etc. All words with the suffix -*itis* denote an inflammatory reaction.

Turmeric is then a natural anti-inflammatory that helps the body to regulate some of the dangerous chronic inflammations. It is well documented that the Indian population suffers fewer cases of cancer per capita than in the United States. This is attributed mainly to their large consumption of spices in their diet. Curry is the most important. A mixture of spices composes it. Turmeric is the key ingredient. This spice gives curry its yellow color.

Although these lower rates of cancer cannot be attributed only to turmeric, as nearly half of the population of India is vegetarian and has a diet rich in legumes and fruits, the statistics are staggering.

An additional piece of information, turmeric, is best absorbed by the body when accompanied by black pepper. A synergy of ingredients.

In a study conducted and published in The Library of Medicine on June 5, 2013, they found that the combination of curcumin, which is the principal ingredient of turmeric, and EGCG, suppresses the growth of cells in lung cancer. This is another great example of the wonderful synergy that exists in natural ingredients. [xii]

Throughout this book, you find I promote natural ingredients, yet I am not one of these people that becomes obsessive with the subject. I do embrace modern medicine when is necessary. A good example is antibiotics. I take them when they are strictly necessary and with a doctor's supervision. So, I don't use them to treat simple viral infections like the common cold.

In my case, I do not wish to go through another bout of cancer treatments, so I help my body fight cancer cells that I know exist, with a diet that is directed to do this job. I am now eating with my brain and not with my stomach.

Ginger.

Another important anti-inflammatory and antioxidant ingredient that is recommended for cancer patients. It helped me during my chemo and radiation sessions to control nausea. A cup of ginger infusion did wonders. A few slices of the root in hot water was all I needed. In a review in Science Direct 2006, on a study done in India, they found that some of the pungent ingredients in ginger had antioxidant and anti-inflammatory effects leading to anti-cancer activity. [xiii]

Chilies

In January 2017,_an article that appeared in the British press reported that chilies could help beat cancer. Researchers found that capsaicin, the principal ingredient, destroys diseased cells. The active ingredient that gives chilies their kick can surround cancer cells and kill them off, which could help develop a cure for cancer. Scientists from Ruhr-University in Bochum, Germany, treated human samples of **breast cancer**, causing apoptosis (cell death) in diseased cells.

Folk medicine has used spices for thousands of years. A study published in the National Library of Medicine documented the antioxidant, anti-inflammatory, and immunomodulatory effects of spices related to the prevention and treatment of several cancers. Including **lung**, liver, breast, stomach, colorectal, cervical, and prostate cancers. The spices mentioned are turmeric, black cumin, ginger, garlic, saffron, black pepper, and chili pepper. [xiv]

CRUCIFEROUS VEGETABLES

Broccoli, Cabbage, Brussels sprouts Kale, Radishes, Watercress, and cauliflower are some examples of these extraordinary vegetables. Apart from being rich in carotenoids, vitamins C, E, and K, folate, and minerals, they provide a group of substances known as glucosinolates. These are Sulphur containing chemicals, which give them their pungent smell and bitter taste. These substances have been found to inhibit the development of cancer in several organs in rats and mice, including the bladder, breast, colon, liver, lung, and stomach. These substances protect against

DNA damage, inactivate carcinogens, cause death in cancer cells, and prevent blood vessels from forming into tumors. [xv]

My favorite legume is broccoli, and I like to "blanch" it in boiling water, leaving the broccoli till it turns bright green. This procedure cooks and kills all external bacteria, keeping the essential nutrients of the legume intact. When cooking legumes or any vegetable, never overcook them, this reduces the essential nutrients that are beneficial to us.

Liliaceae.

This family of plants which includes onions, garlic, shallots asparagus, and aloes, is important in the reduction of nitrosamines and n-nitrous compounds which are harmful substances in charred meat, and nicotine. These plants promote the apoptosis of cancerous cells in the colon, **lung**, breast, prostate, and leukemia. Another important property that this family of plants has, is their ability to balance blood glucose, which benefits patients by reducing the production of insulin and the reduction of glucose in the vessels that feed tumors.

One of my favorite dishes is to air-fry seasonal vegetables with onion, garlic, and asparagus. Once the vegetables are cooked, place them on a bed of basmati rice (low glycemic content) and add curry powder, turmeric, black pepper, chipotle chili powder, and ginger powder. This dish is by itself a bombshell against cancer. It will hold most of the ingredients we have been talking about, and it will help your body fight cancerous cells.

VEGETABLES WITH CAROTENOIDS

Carrots, pumpkins, tomatoes, beetroots, apricots, and most yellow fruits and vegetables. These all contain carotene, a yellow/ orange pigment present in plants serving them in the absorption of light energy for photosynthesis and protecting chlorophyll. In our bodies, dietary carotenoids decrease the risk of disease and certain cancers. The carotenoids that have been studied include beta-carotene, lycopene, lutein, and zeaxanthin. They are strong antioxidants, which help the body eliminate free radicals. Beta-carotene has an added benefit because of its ability to be converted into vitamin A. [xvi]

Many studies show the role that beta-carotene in a pill plays. The studies have focused on lung cancer and the effect this compound has on the metaplasia of bronchial epithelial cells. This change in cells acts as an indicator of the possibility of cancer in the **lung**. The studies show that too much beta-carotene may provoke metaplasia or a modification of cells.

My recommendation is that you should consume this compound in its natural form, as there has been controversy about the dose of pure vitamin A or retinol to treat cancer. Yet, in their natural form, the body seems to take what it needs, and the compounds that accompany these carotenoids act in synergy to make them more efficient.

One of the most important vegetables for cancer is tomatoes. Lycopene, a pigment, gives it its red color. It is a strong compound that fights cancer as an antioxidant. In many studies on animals, researchers have shown that lycopene is an anti-cancer substance, especially for prostate cancer as documented in the Journal of Nutrition 2022. [xvii]

The synergy between tomatoes and broccoli is more powerful than by themselves as their ingredients combined help to protect DNA in our cells. In other studies, researchers found that the body absorbs lycopene much easier with cooked tomatoes.

Soy.

Soy comes in different presentations. Tofu, Tempeh, Dame, soy milk. These are the most common. This legume grows mainly in Asia, where it is widely consumed. This product contains most of the amino acids that the body needs to create protein. The isoflavones, genistein, and daidzein are especially important. In many studies, genistein has been shown to inhibit the growth of cells in breast, prostate, colon, and skin cancer. Daidzein has shown similar properties to cancer.

The isoflavones in soy act as estrogen police in the body. When estrogen levels in women are high, like in premenopausal women, it acts as a blocker so that it cannot affect cells. If estrogen levels are low like in postmenopausal women, it acts as a mild estrogen, copying the functions of estrogen in the body as reported by the Physicians Committee for responsible medicine. [xviii] These functions are important because soy can regulate levels of estrogen, which is the major cause of hormonal-induced cancer. Just be sure that when you buy this product, it's natural and not processed, because then it will lose most of its benefits.

To me, these plants and spices are the most important part of your daily diet. To maintain a healthy fight against cancer, eat as many of these products as possible.

I list other foods that are important to include in your weekly diet below.

Mushrooms.

In Asia, mushrooms form part of their daily diets. They include them in their diets as an additional part of their vegetable intake. Yet their medicinal use has received special attention. Mushrooms such as Shitake, Mitake, Ganoderma Reishi, Coriolus versicolor, Cordyceps sinensis, and Chaga Inonotus have had special attention. In an article published in Huff Post Life, Dr. N. Chiko reported extracts are used to fight cancer and modulate the immune system. [xix]

They are especially important during chemotherapy as they reduce the side effects and protect the kidneys from further damage. The article mentions as a reference over ten studies. In another publication by the National Center for Biotechnology Information, they state medicinal mushrooms represent a growing segment in pharma, because of their incredible amount of bioactive ingredients. [xx]

Other mushrooms which are readily available in the US include Button, Chanterelle, Clamshell, Cremini, King Trumpet, Morel, Oyster, Porcini, and Portobello, all make an incredible meal when eaten with pasta or rice. Be creative and cook them with garlic, a little olive oil, and white wine. They are superb.

Berries.

Strawberries, blueberries, raspberries, and blackberries, among others, have a high content of antioxidants and flavonoids. They contain some of the most important cancer-fighting nutrients, such as Vitamin C, Fiber, Ellagic Acid, Vitamin A, and Folate. All these nutrients together help to eliminate free radicals, which are harmful molecules that affect cells in our bodies.

Another important ingredient in berries and blueberries is resveratrol. Studies have shown that, together with radiation, it is an important deterrent for cells in cervical cancer. A study by Dr. Yujiang Fang, from the University of Missouri-Columbia and reported in the Pathology and Oncology Research, found that when adding blueberry extract to radiation for cervical cancer significantly improves treatment efficacy by nearly 70%. In another study, Dr. Fang found that resveratrol in grapes and blueberries also helped to sensitize cancer cells in the prostate. This sensitization makes cancer cells more vulnerable to radiation treatment.

HERBS AND SPICES

We have spoken of the importance of turmeric, ginger, and chilies as anti-inflammatory agents and cancer-fighting qualities. There are more herbs and spices in your cabinet that are important in the war against cancer. So, do not be afraid to spice your food, all of them will bring an ingredient to the fight. Some of the most commonly used are:

Rosemary.

Two important antioxidant acids are present in this herb. Caffeic and Rosemarinic acid. As we have seen, antioxidants are important in fighting free radicals that harm cells and can induce cancer. Yet the important substances that are found in this herb are carnosol, which hinders tumor development, and terpenes which protect healthy cells during chemotherapy.

Parsley.

Its volatile oil, myristicin, can inhibit tumor formation in the lungs. It also contains apigenin, a natural oil that has been linked to anti-angiogenesis, preventing the formation of blood vessels that feed tumors.

Its strong antibacterial properties are well known. Yet the sulfur compounds found in garlic can block the formation and activation of cancer-forming substances. They enhance the repair of DNA in cells, slowing the reproduction of cancer cells, and provoking apoptosis, or cancer cells' death.

Cayenne.

It comes from the chili pepper family. Its key ingredient, capsaicin, promotes apoptosis in cancer cells. The hotter the chili, the more capsaicin it contains. Capsaicin is important in stopping tumors' growth, and it is especially important to prostate cancer cell destruction.

Cinnamon.

Its active ingredients, cinnamaldehyde, and procyanidin, have been shown that apart from balancing blood sugar in the body, it also is a potent anti-inflammatory agent. Yet in cancer, Cinnamon in recent studies has been shown to stop angiogenesis and block tumor development.

SUPPLEMENTS

Milk Thistle. (*Silybum marianum*)

Its active ingredient, silymarin, has been used for thousands of years throughout Europe as a regenerating stimulant in the liver. It is used to treat cirrhosis and hepatitis. In laboratory studies, it has been shown that it helps chemotherapy drugs against ovarian and **breast cancer**. It also reduces the side effects of some drugs in chemotherapy, stops the growth of cancer cells, and blocks tumor growth.

Saw Palmetto (*Serenoa repens*)

Is the extract of a small palm in the south-eastern states of the US. It is used to treat symptoms of benign prostatic hyperplasia (BPH). In vitro studies, researchers found that Saw Palmetto inhibits the growth of prostate cancer inducing apoptosis of cancer cells, as reported in the National Library of Medicine. [xxi]

It is interesting that in Europe, doctors prescribe Saw Palmetto for BPH, yet the medical community in the USA is still skeptical about its efficacy. This will change as more studies of the extract are done.

Gingko (*Gingko Biloba*)

Traditional medicine in Asia uses Gingko to enhance the amount of oxygen and glucose to reach the brain. There are now a hefty amount of studies worldwide that show that Gingko also has anti-cancer properties. Its phytochemicals stop angiogenesis, provoke cancer cells' apoptosis, are anti-inflammatory, and stabilize DNA mutation. Researchers at Georgetown University Medical Center (2006) have conducted animal experiments where the supplement slowed the growth of tumor growth in **breast cancer**. [xxii]

A study done in Taipei showed that the supplement significantly suppressed cell proliferation by up to 45% in liver cancer as reported in the National Library of Medicine. [xxiii]

A study at the University of Carolina (2008) showed that Gingko Biloba was successful in treating colitis in mice. The study concluded that Gingko was successful in treating colitis and associated colon cancer, also reported in the National Library of Medicine. [xxiv]

Gingko also promotes apoptosis to cancerous cells in the prostate, as established by the journal Hindawi (2019), concluding that the ingredient kaempferol present in Gingko was positive in the treatment of prostate cancer as reported in the National Library of Medicine. [xxv]

Gingko has been well-studied, and highly praised for its ability to promote wellbeing to the human body and its anticancer properties.

Ginseng. (*Panax Ginseng*)

It is the root of a slow-growing plant from the genus *Panax*. The most well-known of these are the Korean ginseng, P. ginseng; South China ginseng, P. notoginseng; American ginseng, P. quinquefolia and Japanese ginseng P. japonicas. This is another well-studied supplement, with incredible properties. Ginseng has long been used in eastern medicine as an adaptogenic substance or a substance that maintains a good balance of the body's functions. (Homeostasis). We use it as an anti-stress substance, stressors being physical, chemical, or biological. It also promotes immune system health. Yet the Korean Ginseng Society (2017) funded several studies published in the National Library of Medicine, where they found that ginseng could suppress tumor growth via different molecular and cellular mechanisms, including the promotion of apoptosis and the activation of immune cells. [xxvi]

An article from the Mayo Clinic (2012) mentions that ginseng can lessen chemotherapy side effects, especially fatigue. This is important to discuss with your doctor, as the principal effect of chemo is fatigue. [xxvii]

In its adaptogenic properties, ginseng balances sugar in the blood, which feeds cancer cells, and balances hormonal homeostasis, preventing spikes that can induce cancer.

Astralagus. (*Astralagus membranaceus*)

This is another adaptogenic supplement that helps to promote immune system functions. It has antiviral properties that are well known to treat the common cold. The polysaccharide in this herb inhibits the proliferation and delays tumor growth in lung and colon cancer, as reported in the National Library of Medicine. [xxviii]

Aloe Vera. (*Aloe vera*)

We all know the properties of this fantastic plant. Naturists use the gel that comes from the fleshy leaves topically for skin ulcers, antimicrobial, and as an antioxidant. It protects you from ultraviolet rays or UV radiation, and in cancer helps skin after radiation therapy. Yet one other benefit, as published in The National Library of Medicine, PubMed.gov (2015), the compounds help apoptosis in breast and cervical cancer cells without affecting normal cells. [xxix]

I used its natural gel from the leaves on my skin as I received radiation. It helped reduce considerably the burn of radiation. I talked it over with my radiation oncologist; he was very open-minded about it and determined that it would not affect the protocol of radiation that was diagnosed for me.

Dark Chocolate

In an article by the National Foundation for Cancer Research (2016) the author promotes the use of dark chocolate, 70% cocoa, for cancer prevention. Its high content of flavonoids, and antioxidants, helps the body fight toxic residue in our bodies. The article does mention that it also contains unhealthy saturated fat that can raise bad cholesterol levels. So, the consumption should be in small portions. xxx

I have only listed a few supplements I use and feel comfortable mentioning. There are many more and you should discuss using all supplements during treatment with your doctors. Most times, they will prefer you not to use any supplements during chemotherapy. This is understandable, as they are not specialists in nutritional supplements, and they would rather not include another variable in the complex treatment of chemotherapy. During treatment, always talk to your doctor. I started using these supplements after treatment, and only when I was sure that they will not interfere with medicines that were prescribed post-treatment.

GUT HEALTH

There has been a lot of attention recently in the media on Gut Health. Researchers have published studies, and the public is paying attention to their gut health. What it means is that we should try to keep a good balance between good bacteria and bad bacteria.

There are more bacteria in our bodies than cells. Some concentrate on the GI Track. The Gut Microbiome helps to digest our food and turn it into nutrients the body can absorb. It also maintains the immune system's health and mental health.

Cancer treatment, be it chemotherapy, radiation, or surgery, affects our Gut Microbiome, allowing bad bacteria to proliferate. These bacteria create havoc in our bodies, affecting our general wellbeing. What is interesting is that researchers have proved that cancer treatment and radiation directly affect our gut bacteria, reducing our ability to fight our disease this was reported in two articles in the National Library of Medicine. [xxxi] [xxxii]

In 2007, doctors knew little of the Gut Microbiome. My doctors, although they were specialists on the GI track, never explained this important factor to me. The result was that I suffered debilitating cramps and chronic diarrhea, with its dehydrating consequences, for many years. Doctors diagnosed my symptoms as IBS (irritable bowel syndrome). What it meant is that they could not pinpoint the real problem, so they just wrapped it up in the general area of IBS. Something they do too often.

I was lucky to stumble on a Functional Medical article four years later that talked about the balance of the gut microbiome and the general health of the body. This was an eye-opener. I went into a treatment of probiotics and prebiotics, together with a high-fiber diet, and in two weeks I saw promising results. (I had avoided high-fiber foods thinking they caused my problem.)

If you go through any of the conventional treatments, please talk to your doctor regarding a probiotic and prebiotic treatment, it will save you a lot of miserable side effects like cramps, diarrhea, depression, and anxiety, plus it will boost your immune system that is so important to fight our disease.

SUMMARY

Regarding nutrition, it is important to prepare for treatment. Maintain a good diet, eat well, and exercise. Your body must be strong and ready for the treatments, be it chemotherapy, radiation, or/and surgery. These are huge stressors to the body. Prepare your body to be strong before all treatments. Before my treatment, I went to my brother's house on the seaside, and I would go for long walks to prepare my mind and my body, eating super healthy food. Zero alcohol, zero tobacco, and zero sugar, for ten days. When I went back home, I was ready for whatever was thrown at me. I felt good about my body and how clean it had become.

During treatments for chemotherapy and radiation, it is important to maintain a good routine of eating, exercising, and working. Eat as much vegetables as you can and keep a healthy weight. This will help your immune system to stay in optimal condition.

The worst enemy of treatment is an infection. So, stay away from people with infections, especially children, do not handshake, and sanitize your hands with antibacterial gel as

202 | LAWRENCE W DICKINS

much as possible. Clean telephones, keypads, remote controls, steering wheels, and light switches as much as possible. They are tremendous sources of bacteria.

All supplement intake during treatment MUST be supervised by your doctor.

Eat as many natural foods as possible. Get your team to do the shopping and avoid all processed foods.

The macronutrients you should include in the meals that give you energy are carbohydrates, fibers, fats, proteins, and water.

The micronutrients your body needs are present in the natural foods you consume. You don't need vitamin supplements unless your doctor recommends them. There will be moments when a boost of vitamin C or A might be necessary. Also, an increase in mineral iron if your doctor perceives anemia.

My recommendation of foods herbs, teas, and spices that are good for cancer cell destruction are Green Tea, Turmeric, Ginger, Cruciferous Veggies (Broccoli, Cauliflower, Cabbage etc.), Liliaceae Vegetables (garlic Onion, etc.,), Carotenoids Vegetables (Carrots, Pumpkin, Tomatoes, etc.), Soy, Mushrooms, Berries, Cold-Water Fish (Salmon, Sardines, etc.) and dark chocolate. Supplements that I started using after treatment include Milk Thistle, Saw Palmetto, Echinacea, Gingko Biloba, Astralagus, Ginseng, and Aloe Vera.

Chemo, radiation, and antibiotics affect our gut health. Check with your doctor whether you should take probiotics or prebiotics to counteract these effects.

CHAPTER SEVEN

"Opportunities multiply as they are seized"
—Sun Tzu **The Art of War**

DEALING WITH RECURRENCE

When cancer returns, it can be distressing for you and your loved ones. The medical evaluation is challenging, and all the feelings you felt when you were originally diagnosed may reemerge, or perhaps be even stronger this time around. You may feel more cautious, guarded, and pessimistic than you ever have. You may be dissatisfied with your body and with your cancer treatment team. The recurrence of cancer raises several difficulties and questions. Here are some of the most prevalent:

Was there anything I could have done to prevent the recurrence?

Numerous individuals blame themselves for missing a medical appointment, eating improperly, or delaying blood work or imaging tests. But even if everything is done correctly, cancer might recur.

Even with our current understanding of how cancer develops and spreads, it remains in many ways a mystery.

Why me?

Looking for an answer to "Why me?" can cause restless nights and intense introspection for some individuals. Others believe that it does not matter why something has occurred; what matters is how to best cope with it.

Anxiety can sap a person's energy, which is necessary for coping with the condition. If you are unable to go past this question, consult with your cancer care team. You may require an introduction to a mental health expert who may assist you in overcoming these emotions.

On the other hand, when I was diagnosed the second time, it was a moment of reflection. I knew that my old lifestyle was not helping me. So, I entered treatments with renewed determination that this was going to be the last time I would face this disease. I changed my whole lifestyle, my nutrition, my way of thinking and added an exercise regime. This I did with discipline and conviction.

Recurrence and cancer treatment

If the cancer returns, your physician will discuss treatment options and the likelihood of success for each.

Ensure that you comprehend the purpose of each potential treatment. Is it for cancer control? Is it a remedy? Is it to improve your comfort? You may also elect to obtain a second opinion or seek treatment at a cancer center with more expertise in your particular form of cancer.

Typically, clinical trials are also made available to patients with cancer recurrence. If you're considering participating in a clinical trial, you'll want to know its purpose and likelihood of helping you.

Please keep in mind that it is crucial to verify your insurance coverage alongside the medical treatment options you are considering.

Why can't I receive the same treatment for the recurrence as I did for the initial diagnosis?

Some individuals end up receiving some of the same cancer treatments they had for their first diagnosis. For instance, a woman with recurrent lung cancer may need further surgery to remove the tumor. She may also undergo radiation therapy, particularly if it has not been administered previously. Her physician and she may then consider chemotherapy and/or hormone therapy.

Consider, too, that cancer cells can develop resistance to chemotherapy. Returning cancers frequently do not react as well to treatment as the first ones did.

Another reason your doctor may choose a different treatment is the possibility of negative effects. Certain chemotherapy medications, for instance, might cause cardiac difficulties and nerve damage in the hands and feet. Continued administration of this medication could exacerbate your symptoms or cause long-term negative effects.

Ask your cancer care team why they propose a particular course of treatment for your recurrence at this time. Discuss your alternatives with your team, members of your support group, and, most importantly, your family.

Scientists are investigating genetic testing that may predict the likelihood of recurrence of malignancies such as lung, breast, colon, and melanoma. Some formulas can be used to assess the likelihood of recurrence for certain cancer types. However, even with such predictions, recurrence uncertainty cannot be avoided. This is one reason why recurrence is so difficult to manage. There are no guarantees that can be relied upon.

How to determine if you should continue treatment

There is no singular response to this question. It depends on the type of cancer, how it is affecting you, what your cancer care team tells you, and how you and your family feel about the situation. During cancer treatment, you are under the care of a physician, the progression of the cancer is slowed, and side effects and symptoms are monitored and treated. For some, receiving cancer treatment makes them feel better and stronger because they are actively fighting the disease. For some, treatment has the opposite effect; it may make them feel more exhausted or less liberated. You alone determine how you will live your life. You'll also want to know how your family feels about it. Their feelings are crucial since they are experiencing cancer alongside you. However, keep in mind that the final decision rests with you.

Regardless of whether you desire cancer treatment, you should always receive supportive or palliative care. It is not anticipated that this treatment will cure cancer or prolong life. Even if there is little chance of curing the cancer, the care focuses on making the patient's life as well as possible.

Treatment is administered even though a cure is not anticipated. For many patients, this method can control cancer for years. The goal of treatment is to shrink the tumor, alleviate symptoms, and prolong life. Even though it can be challenging, many families adapt to this treatment schedule.

Coping emotionally with recurrence.

When cancer returns, not everyone has the same emotions and thoughts. And not everyone has the answers provided here, but many have similar concerns and questions.

Placing blame

"I'm so angry and distressed! Cancer had vanished! These are meant to be my golden years of retirement. Now I face more treatment. It is entirely the fault of my doctor."

It is understandable to be extremely upset when the reverse of what was anticipated occurs. The last thing anyone anticipates is having to undergo additional cancer treatment they believed to be eradicated. It is normal to want to assign blame. The obvious choice is your physician. After all, this is the physician who diagnosed you as cancer-free on your initial visit.

During your initial treatment, you may have felt that something was done improperly. Perhaps you feel that your physician did not follow up with you closely enough. Or you may feel that you were not listened to as attentively as you believe you should have been. Regardless of your emotions, they must be addressed immediately. There are steps you can take to resolve any issues you are currently facing. You may wish to discuss your concerns with your physician. Try to resolve any negative feelings you may have regarding your treatment.

It is highly unlikely that a doctor would intentionally fail to provide optimal care on the initial visit. When you think about it, that makes absolutely no sense. Your doctors want you to succeed; this contributes to their success. But if you cannot work with your current physician, it may be prudent to find a new one. You may find that a fresh start with a new cancer care team improves your outlook and makes you feel better about your current circumstances.

Anger

It is natural to feel angry and sad about a cancer recurrence, and you may need support and someone to talk to about these emotions. There are various sources for this type of assistance. For some, their support group serves as their house of worship. Others may benefit from a formal support group or an online support group. Other cancer survivors who have experienced recurrence are uniquely able to comprehend and offer support. Still, some individuals prefer private one-on-one counseling. Request a referral from your friends, family, or a physician you respect. Ensure that you have a means of expressing your emotions. You are worthy of being heard.

Depression and nervousness

People who are suffering from a cancer recurrence frequently experience some degree of despair and worry. But when a person is emotionally distressed for an extended period or has difficulty with day-to-day tasks, they may be suffering from depression or severe anxiety that requires medical intervention. These issues can cause significant distress and make it difficult to adhere to a treatment program.

Even if you are clinically depressed or anxious, you still have a few advantages.

- Depression is treatable, and most treatments are effective.
- Improving your physical symptoms and acting may help improve your mood.
- You have fought cancer before and have gained valuable knowledge. Try the things that helped you previously. Those same relationships and coping skills could be beneficial now.

Family and friends should be on the lookout for signs of distress. If they observe symptoms of depression or anxiety, they should encourage the individual to seek professional help. Anxiety and clinical depression can be treated with a variety of methods, such as medication, psychotherapy, or both. These treatments can help an individual feel better and enhance their quality of life.

Hopelessness

There are various ways to view and discuss cancers that have returned. Is there a possibility that you may not survive the recurrence of your cancer? Yes. Does this imply that there is no hope? No. When cancer returns, you may find that your expectations differ completely from when you were initially diagnosed.

There is no doubt that the situation is graver if cancer has returned, but for many patients, this merely means that their therapy will be different and possibly more severe than before. You must communicate with your cancer care team. They can provide you with a solid indication of what to expect. There is a possibility your cancer cannot be cured, but there are measures that can be taken to prevent it from spreading. You and your family must understand the purpose of any treatment.

MANAGEMENT OF CANCER AS A CHRONIC DISEASE

Cancer is not usually a singular occurrence. Cancer can be properly monitored and treated, but it is occasionally incurable. It can be a chronic ailment, similar to diabetes or cardiovascular disease. This is frequently the case with ovarian cancer, lung cancer, chronic leukemia, and some lymphomas. Sometimes cancers that have moved to other parts of the body or returned, such as metastatic breast or prostate cancer, also become chronic.

The cancer may be managed by treatment, meaning it may appear to disappear or remain unchanged. As long as you're receiving treatment, the cancer might not develop or spread. When treatment shrinks the cancer, it is sometimes possible to take a vacation until the cancer begins to grow again. In any instance, however, the cancer remains; it does not vanish and does not remain eradicated; it has not been treated.

Living with cancer is distinct from surviving cancer. And it is becoming more prevalent daily.

How is chronic cancer described?

A physician may use the phrase controlled if tests or scans indicate that the disease is stable over time. Such cancers are continuously monitored to ensure that they do not progress.

The recurrence and remission cycle

The majority of chronic cancers are incurable, but others can be managed for months or even years. In actuality, there is always a possibility that cancer will enter remission. With everyday new treatments, this is a fact. There are several sorts of remission.

- A complete response or complete remission occurs when a treatment eradicates all tumors that can be measured or detected by a diagnostic test.

- A partial response or partial remission indicates that cancer partially reacted to treatment but did not completely disappear. A partial response is most typically characterized as at least a 50% reduction in a measurable tumor. In this context, remission often refers to partial remission.

To qualify as either a form of remission, the absence of a tumor or reduction in tumor size must persist for a minimum of one month. Since there is no way to predict how long a remission would remain, remission does not necessarily indicate that the cancer has been cured.

Certain malignancies, such as ovarian cancer, have an inherent inclination toward recurrence and remission. This repeated pattern of growth, shrinkage, and stabilization can frequently result in long-term survival during which the cancer can be managed as a chronic condition. Treatment can be used to control cancer, alleviate symptoms, and extend life expectancy.

Progression

Stable cancers may be referred to as stable diseases. The process by which cancer grows spreads, or worsens is known as cancer progression. When cancer returns from remission, it is said to have advanced. In chronic malignancies, recurrence and progression can mean essentially the same thing.

Progression may indicate that you must recommence treatment to bring the cancer back into remission. If the cancer progresses during or shortly after treatment, a change in therapy may be necessary.

When the treatment fails to eradicate all cancer cells, progression and recurrence occur. Even if the majority of cancer cells were eliminated, some were either unaffected or able to adapt sufficiently to survive the treatment. These cancer cells can then develop and divide sufficiently to reappear on diagnostic testing.

Treating chronic cancer.

The majority of individuals are willing to do whatever to treat cancer, whether it's the first therapy or the second or third. Your physician will discuss your treatment options with you. You may also elect to seek a second opinion or undergo treatment at a comprehensive cancer center with more expertise in your particular form of cancer. Additionally, there may be clinical studies accessible.

Some people receive the same sorts of treatment they had the first time (such as surgery or chemotherapy), but as cancer develops, some treatments may become less effective. Treatment decisions are dependent on the type of disease, the location of the cancer, the amount of cancer, the extent of its spread, your overall health, and your personal preferences.

Chemotherapy

Cancers are often treated with chemotherapy (chemo) in one of two methods over the long term.

- Chemotherapy is administered regularly to keep the cancer under control. This is also known as maintenance chemotherapy. This may help prevent the spread of disease and prolong survival.
- Chemotherapy may also be administered just when the cancer reactivates. Imaging and blood tests are used to monitor the malignancy, and chemo is administered if the disease progresses.

Consider, too, that cancer cells can develop resistance to chemotherapy. Frequently, recurring cancers do not react as effectively to treatment as the first tumors did. For instance, if the cancer returns within a year or two of receiving chemotherapy, it may be resistant to this type of chemotherapy, and an alternative treatment may be more effective. Sometimes doctors would suggest, "Since you've already taken this medication, we must try another." This may indicate that doctors believe you have received the maximum benefit from a particular type of drug and that a new drug will probably be more effective at killing cancer cells since it operates differently.

Sometimes, your doctor will not prescribe a particular medication due to the risk of a certain adverse effect or because you have already taken it. Some chemotherapy medications, for instance, can cause cardiac difficulties or nerve damage in the hands and feet. To keep giving you that same drug would risk making those problems worse or maybe lead to permanent damage.

Making therapeutic decisions

Ask your doctor why he or she recommends a particular course of treatment at this time. Do you have two or three treatment choices? Determine what you may anticipate from each treatment. Discuss these options with your cancer care team, members of your support group, and your family in particular. Then you can pick the optimal choice for yourself.

Therapy lengths.

This is an excellent question; however, it is quite difficult to answer. There is no way to specify a precise time restriction. Depending on your circumstances and a few other things, the answer could be:

- The type of cancer you have.
- The treatment schedule or plan.
- The length of time between cancer recurrences.
- The aggressiveness of the cancer cell type.
- Your age.
- Your overall health.
- The way you tolerate treatment.
- How well the cancer responds to treatment.
- The types of treatment you receive.

Chronic cancer can be difficult to manage because there are no promises that can be relied upon. Discuss any questions or concerns with your physician and the rest of your cancer treatment team. They are the most familiar with your situation and may give you an idea of what to expect.

Cancer survival.

The initial months of cancer treatment are a period of transition. But when you're living with persistent cancer, you may feel stuck in this change — you don't know what to expect or what will happen next.

Living with cancer is less about "returning to normal" than it is about discovering your new normal. People frequently claim that life now has fresh significance or that they view things differently. Every day has a fresh significance.

Your new "normal" may involve modifying the way you eat, the activities you engage in, and your support system. It may necessitate scheduling cancer treatments around work and vacation time. It will necessitate integrating treatment into your daily routine; you may require treatment for the rest of your life.

Repeated recurrences, frequently accompanied by shorter intervals between remissions, can be disheartening and stressful. Even more discouraging would be if the cancer never disappeared. The question of whether or not to continue treating recurring or persistent cancer is a valid one. Your decisions regarding continued therapy are individualized and depend on your requirements, desires, and capabilities. There is no right or incorrect way to manage this period of illness.

Nonetheless, it is essential to understand that even those who are not cured of cancer may continue to survive for months or years, albeit with alterations to their lives. Numerous families adapt to this therapy program.

Cancer that cannot be cured does not preclude hope or assistance; you may live with a disease that may be treated and controlled for a considerable period.

Living with uncertainty

Here are some suggestions that have helped people feel more positive and cope with the persistent uncertainty and anxiety of cancer:

- Be informed. Find out what you can do now to improve your health and what services are available to you and your loved ones. This can help you feel more in control.
- Recognize that you lack control over certain parts of your cancer. It is beneficial to accept something rather than resist it.
- Recognize your fears, but practice overcoming them. It's natural for these thoughts to enter your head, but you don't need to dwell on them. Some imagine them drifting away or vanishing into thin air. Others give them over to a higher authority for management. Regardless of how you choose to let go, doing so can save you from wasting time and energy needlessly worrying.
- Communicate your sentiments of worry or apprehension to a trustworthy friend or counselor. Many people feel less anxious and are better able to

appreciate each day because of being honest about their feelings. People have discovered that when people express intense emotions, such as rage and fear, they are better able to let go of them. It's difficult to consider and articulate one's emotions. If cancer is dominating your life, it may be beneficial to find a means to express your emotions.

- Focus on the now rather than the uncertain future or the unpleasant past. If you can find a way to be peaceful inside yourself, even for a few minutes a day, you can start to recall that peace when other things are happening—when life is busy, scary, and confusing.

- Make time for your true desires. You may find yourself contemplating the things you've always wanted to accomplish but never found the time. It is acceptable to pursue these things, but don't forget to appreciate simple pleasures and have fun.

- Pursue a positive outlook, which might help you feel better about life, even if a remedy is unavailable. Almost everyone may discover reasons to be grateful or optimistic. But do not attempt to be constantly cheery and optimistic; nobody is! You must pay attention to all of your emotions, even the "bad" ones. You are permitted to have unpleasant days, feel sad or angry, or grieve as necessary.

- Use your energy to concentrate on what you can do today to maintain optimal health. Make healthful modifications to your diet and your exercise routine.

- Find ways to unwind and enjoy alone and social time.
- Be as physically active as possible. Communicate with your cancer care team with your realistic expectations.

Control what is possible. Some claim that organizing their lives makes them feel less anxious. Controllable factors include being involved in your health care, attempting to find your "new normal," and making changes to your lifestyle. Even establishing a regular regimen can empower you. And while no one can control their every thought, some claim they have chosen not to focus on fearful ones.

Grief

It is normal to feel depressed upon learning that cancer cannot be cured. Even if you know there is a good chance you will live a long time with cancer, this sadness may persist. You may experience grief over the loss of what you believed to be your future. This is difficult to manage without emotional support.

Grief can have physical, emotional, and mental effects on a person. It can hinder day-to-day activities. It takes time and effort to adjust to these significant life changes. Many individuals find it beneficial to have friends with whom they can discuss these issues. If you cannot think of anyone, you may want to consider finding a counselor or support group.

Dealing with melancholy

Depression and anxiety are frequently experienced by those coping daily with cancer. But when a person is emotionally distressed for an extended period and has difficulty with day-to-day activities, they may require medical attention for depression or severe anxiety. These issues can cause significant distress and make it difficult to enjoy life and adhere to a treatment plan.

Even if you are clinically depressed or anxious, there are a few positives:

- Depression is frequently treatable, and treatment is typically effective.
- Improving your physical symptoms and taking action will probably help improve your mood.

Anxiety and depression can be treated with a variety of methods, such as medication, psychotherapy, or both. These treatments can help an individual feel better and enhance their quality of life.

Getting support

Any form of support enables you to discuss your emotions and develop coping skills. Many people who participate in support groups have a higher quality of life, including improved sleep and appetite, according to studies.

A support group can be an effective resource for patients and their families. Talking with others in similar circumstances can help alleviate feelings of isolation. Those who have shared similar experiences may provide you with helpful insights. At the end of the book, I list several support groups you can contact.

Types of Assistance

There are numerous types of support programs, including individual therapy, group counseling, and support groups.

Counseling. You may benefit from a personal relationship with a counselor who can provide you with individual attention and encouragement. It is essential to locate a counselor with expertise and experience in caring for cancer patients. Your cancer care team is the best resource for locating local counselors.

Support groups. Some support groups are formal and emphasize cancer education or emotion management. Others are social and casual. Some clubs consist only of cancer patients or caretakers, while others include spouses, family members, and friends. Other organizations concentrate on specific cancer types or disease stages. The duration of group meetings might range from a predetermined number of weeks to an ongoing program. Some sessions are closed to new members, while others welcome walk-ins.

You must obtain information about any cancer support group you are considering joining to ensure that there are patients in all phases of therapy, including those whose illness is incurable. Ask the group leader or facilitator about the types of patients in the group and whether anyone is suffering from persistent cancer.

Online support groups may also be a viable alternative. I have listed some support groups at the end of the book.

Religion and spirituality

For some people, religion can be a source of strength. During a cancer diagnosis, some find new faith. Others find that cancer reinforces their existing faith or provides them with newfound strength. If you are religious, a minister, rabbi, other religious leader, or pastoral counselor can assist you in identifying your spiritual needs and locating spiritual support. Some clergy members are specially trained to assist cancer patients and their families.

Even among those who do not practice traditional religion, spirituality is important too. Many people are comforted by the realization that they are a part of something greater than themselves, which can assist them in discovering their life's purpose. Some individuals benefit from practicing forgiveness or performing modest acts of kindness. Others cater to their spiritual needs by meditating, spending time in nature, or practicing appreciation, to name just a few of the numerous ways they do so.

If it is difficult for you to find meaning in your life or make peace with yourself, you may wish to spend time with a reputable counselor or member of the clergy who can assist you with this crucial task.

Members of the family and loved ones.

You may be concerned about how your illness and treatment will affect your loved ones. This is a difficult trip to do alone, and everyone needs assistance and support from their loved ones. It's difficult to know where to begin, who to speak with, and what to say. Several books will help you face this dilemma.

Questions for your oncology team

- How long do you believe I will survive this cancer? What is the range of survival times for individuals in my predicament?
- How will I know if my cancer is worsening?
- What do you believe I should anticipate at this time?
- What symptoms should I monitor and report to you?
- How frequently will I require therapy or visit the doctor?
- What is the current objective of treatment? Control of the disease? Comfort?
- What tests will I need to monitor for cancer progression?
- What treatments are available for my symptoms (pain, fatigue, nausea, etc.)?
- Am I able to join any support groups?
- How will I pay for my medical care? Will it be covered by my health insurance?

Hope

Most people view cancer as an illness that people contract, have treatment for, and either recover from or die from. When cancer is first diagnosed, a cure is hoped for. And for some individuals, this possibility exists. But many cancer patients are treated but are not cured; they live with cancer. Hope is something that all cancer patients need to have. When you are diagnosed with cancer, a whole world opens in the realm of all possibilities. Living with cancer is one of them. So, if your mind is focused on winning this battle, you are helping your body to do so.

SUMMARY

Recurrence is a troubling circumstance. The mind searches for explanations, shifting from blaming oneself to blaming others.

Cancer recurrence is treated similarly to the initial diagnosis of cancer. However, tests must be conducted to determine if the medications that put you into remission are still effective or if different medications must be administered. Be certain to comprehend each treatment and its repercussions, as your mind must be prepared and resolved to enter a new phase of therapy. Remember that your mental condition is essential to fighting this sickness. There is a possibility that you will have to decide whether to continue therapy. This is a highly personal choice, and I cannot assist you. Nevertheless, if there is a glimmer of hope that you may achieve remission, I believe you are worthy of the treatments.

Managing cancer as a chronic disease is difficult, and the mind plays a significant role once again. Learning to live with a chronic illness is life-changing and must be dealt with.

Like diabetics, you accept your treatments in stride and continue with your life.

The cycles of remission and recurrence vary, but treatments will control the malignancy, alleviate symptoms, and lengthen survival time. Living with cancer involves finding your new self. Your new life and its new significance. It is futile to consider your former self or others; this is who you are now, and you will find the strength to continue living with this condition. Seek help from loved ones or support groups.

There is a list of questions you should ask your oncologist, but please note that the answers are estimations, so take them with a grain of salt and decide how you will make your future.

CHAPTER EIGHT

"If the mind is willing, the flesh can go on and on without many things."
— Sun Tzu, The Art of War

SIXTH STEP

THE POWER OF THE MIND

On the 19 of October 2007, doctors discharged me from the hospital. Doctors, nurses, and hospital assistants went by my room to say goodbye and wish me good luck. My family and team were there with me thanking all the staff for a well-made job, and all their kindness and professionalism. We had wrestled with chemotherapy, radiation, surgery, and pulmonary infection. It elated everybody except me.

After having spent three months in the hospital and going through all the treatments and being sedated for over 20 days, I got used to a routine. They fed, bathed, and looked after me all the time. They fed me through a tube directly into my intestine and hydrated me intravenously. I could take small steps to the bathroom. That was all.

Going back home was attractive for obvious reasons, yet I was scared. I would have to take care of myself, and I did not know if I was ready. Everybody was very supportive, but I understood that all my team was eager to get on with their own lives. My body had gone through a lot of traumas and mentally, I was exhausted. The only thing I knew was that I was not the same and that I could not do things I used to do. My biggest test was still to come.

After surgery, my oncologist prescribed another round of chemotherapy to kill any remaining cancer cells that could have escaped during surgery. This chemo I could do as an outpatient. That meant that I would go for a round of chemo in the doctor's office and then get back home. They delivered the chemo through a portable infusion pump; a cylindrical tube that, by pressure, fed the liquid directly to the port in my chest. After the first week, we got to a routine of my visits to the doctor's office in the hospital. Although, most of the time I was alone, and this gave me a lot of time to think.

My first aim was to get well or at least sufficiently well to work again. I did some exercise, mainly walking up and down in the house. I concentrate on my diet. Now this was another ballgame. I had lost 22 pounds in the hospital and was now weighing a mere 121 pounds! I had to add some weight and elevate my calorie intake. This was easily said. I did not count on the fact that my gastrointestinal system had changed, and I suffered severe "dumping." [1] The situation

---

[1] A syndrome where food passes through the stomach into the

was that the surgeon formed my stomach into a tube attached to my larynx as an esophageal duct. I was not digesting properly. These 'dumping' syndromes accompanied by serious cramps kept me doubled in bed for long hours. Another obstacle was that after a time the "anastomosis" [2] between my stomach and larynx, kept on closing because of scar tissue. So, I had to undergo an endoscopy to open the passage. In the beginning, this happened nearly every week. Between chemotherapy, dumping, cramps, and endoscopies, I was exhausted.

My doctors could not help me as they informed me that each case was different, although they helped with the pain caused by cramps. I looked for help in esophageal cancer forums and see what some patients recommend, and what types of foods they were consuming to keep some nutrients. The information was very disappointing. Everybody was different and dealt with their problems differently. In one case one guy even recommended I should drink beer, not only because it was nutritious, but that it also helped him to burp easier! I then gave that forum up, and I had to resort to the old fashion way. Trial and error.

This way I was conscious of what I put in my mouth every moment of my life. I kept a simple record of foods that could stay in my system for longer than three hours, and foods that were rejected immediately.

---

intestines directly and expelled immediately.
[2] A surgical connection between two tubular structures

Not everything was as easy, as the shadow of depression kept on appearing and making things more difficult; making me question if all this was worth it most of the time. Somehow determination would alternate with depression as I went into my third month being home. It was difficult. I would get up every morning and hope that whatever I put in my mouth I could keep enough time in my organism to extract some nutrients and give me some energy. If I could not keep them, between nausea and fatigue I had to look for alternatives. Slowly I found some foods that helped me. I could retain pasta but not whole grain as the fiber affected my bowel movement (or so I thought), skinless chicken, lean beef, and some cooked vegetables.

Despair took me to anger, anger took me to resolution, and resolution took me to determination. I had to control my mind and my body somehow. This was hard, as I thought that after going through all the treatments and surgeries, my life would just pick up where I left it. That was not the case.

So, the first thing I learned was to listen to my internal voice.

YOUR MIND AS AN INSTRUMENT

Most of us spend a lifetime going through life without ever putting any attention to our thought process: what the mind thinks, what it fears, what it needs, and what it thinks about itself. We ignore the most important process of our existence.

Fear is one of those obstacles that we live with, and yet some of us just permit it to exist in our lives without trying to analyze why it exists and how we can manage it. The fear of cancer is a feeling that creeps into our minds, and if we let it, can lead us into depression and too many negative thoughts of this illness.

At one point, we must face our fear. The sooner the better. If you avoid it, you cannot move forward, and you will become anxious. We must find a way to achieve personal control, and we can achieve it by focusing on the things that we can control and letting go of the things that we can't.

"God, grant me the serenity to accept the things I cannot change, the courage to change the things I can, and the wisdom to know the difference." [3]

Fear takes us to focus on the negative things in our lives and reinforces our anxieties. Yet we can do something about it. We can start focusing on the positive things in our lives. Joy, and a general good feeling about life, the people we love, the laughter of children at sunrise. There are so many things

---

[3] Reinhold Neibuhr

we can be thankful for, and if we focus our attention on these, fear and anxiety will dissipate.

Guilt and self-worth are other feelings that creep in while battling cancer. The question we make ourselves about the fact that are things worth it, or what did I do to deserve this? Or even worse, I shouldn't have done this or that. These are all self-doubt questions that should not have a place in our minds. We can eradicate this by finding a true purpose. Something that will give you the strength to go on. In my case, one day I decided I was going to win this battle. Whatever it took. I shared this with my loved ones, and the hope and strength in their eyes gave me purpose.

When things got bad, and they did, I would take long walks in nature, and I would calm my mind by just thinking about the beauty of life and my surroundings.

If you feel disconnected and cannot find any relief, please get support. Not only from family, but look for professional help, or join a forum for your specific cancer, and share your experience. It will surprise you at how great it feels. It's like the dumping of a burden that you alone have been carrying. At the end of the book, I will give you links and telephones to support groups in the USA, Canada, and the UK.

Battling fear and anxiety is one of the most important steps to take to beat cancer. Once you have control of your mind, you can do anything, and mind over matter will be one of them.

As human beings, we are creatures of habit. The mind is the same. What you practice is what you are. So be careful about what you practice. Here we shall practice positive thinking. Not that everything is wonderful, but in the good things that surround us. These are the thoughts that will give us energy and strength and will constantly dominate our minds.

We constantly forget that to change something outside ourselves, the first step is to change something inside us. To change things like paradigms and beliefs, it will be necessary to train our mind to have only thought of success, and freedom from our illness, nullifying completely all negative thoughts that only feed our doubts and fears.

We must maintain our mind "consciously" or deliberately occupied with positive thoughts, training our mind "muscles" to only think of a positive outcome.

VISUALIZATION

One technique that fights cancer is by visualizing an outcome. Visualization is a mental rehearsal of an outcome. You create images in your mind of having or doing whatever you want. You then repeat these images for some ten minutes over and over every day, imagining a desired result. The key to successful visualization is to visualize a successful result. You must trick your mind into thinking that you have already achieved what you desire, instead of hoping something that you desire will happen or that you expect a successful outcome. The subconscious mind is the target of this. Your conscious mind will know that you are only exercising, yet your subconscious mind will take it as a fact. The subconscious mind will then act upon the images you have created, whether they reflect reality or not.

The more you practice this, the better you will get in using all your senses in this way. Smell, taste, hearing, and touch, are all focused on one outcome.

In my first phase of chemotherapy in July 2007, I read about visualization in the hospital's library. I was extremely skeptical about many things that were not scientifically proven. My education had made me stricter in my beliefs, especially in things that had to do with medical matters. Yet I gave it a go. I had nothing to lose. During the long hours of chemotherapy, I would close my eyes and just visualize my cancer cells being destroyed. I would smell the chemicals, feel the drugs going into my cancer, and hear the battle of the destruction of cancer cells. I did this throughout my chemotherapy cycle, so after a time, it became a habit.

I cannot prove the results. But when doctors performed a CT scan, my tumor had disappeared completely. The doctors attributed this to a successful radiation and chemotherapy treatment, but a daunting question persisted in my mind. Why didn't the treatment work in 2003 when the cancer first appeared? I will not have a definite answer. The fact is that as I write these lines; I have been in remission for 15 years.

During my treatment, certain nutritional habits had changed, and these could have also had some effect on the result. If everything I did helped to eradicate cancer from my system, great, I would do it again without a doubt.

During visualization, I also used neurolinguistics.

The science is called Neuro-linguistic programming (NPL) and is used by coaches to improve communication and change behavior. It connects three elements: neurology relating to the brain and the nervous system. Linguistics, or the use and effect of language we use. Programming is the behaviors that are used to achieve a goal. It is based on the theory that language can change behavior when the brain uses and process it. What is important to know is that, as with visualization, we must consciously use language to change the perception of cancer in our subconscious. We need this as we all know that cancer is not an easy fight, yet through NLP we can change that perception and make a positive impact on our attitude towards the results of the treatment. I would use a mantra when I was imagining the battle of cells in my body and the destruction of cancerous cells. I would repeat to myself, "I going to win" "I am going to beat cancer". This made me positive about my fight, and it would strengthen my resolution to beat this disease. It also strengthened me, as I would not let my guard down in my resolution, and even when I was feeling fatigued by the drugs, my mind was still fighting and pushing my body to do the same.

INTERNAL VOICE

So, the way we perceive cancer is important. The way we perceive it will determine not only what decisions we make but also the way our body will attack it. If you see it as an illness that has taken possession of your life, then it will, and everything will move around it. Notwithstanding all the effort you put into the fight, it will still dominate your life.

If we think about it, cancer is a phenomenon that appears in our bodies. Multiple factors, internal and external, dictate its appearance. All these factors together make cancer cells appear and multiply without control.

Yet what happens when we take control of those factors? What happens if, instead of aiding the proliferation of these cells in our body, we limit them by conscious actions? Well, simply the cells would not proliferate and probably not even appear. Well then, this is the first thing we must do in our fight against cancer. We must take control of our lives and our body. Yet this time with a new objective to eradicate this illness from our bodies, and to strengthen our immune system to maintain a healthy balance between our bodies and our environment.

In the last years of research, modern medicine has dedicated itself to finding formulas and drugs to attack the cancerous cell and kill it. Hence the treatments of chemotherapy and radiology, which do exactly that, killing cancer cells, and as a collateral effect killing healthy cells too. Unfortunately, to date, there is still no other way to do it successfully, on a cheaper and massive scale. Yes, there have been specific studies to kill certain types of cancers, yet this is still the most efficient way.

Fortunately, modern medicine has started a new focus on fighting this disease. Now the scientific world is focusing not on the cell itself, but on the environment this cell exists. What does it feed on? How does the cell get its nutrients? How does it multiply? What is the preferred medium of existence? All this gives scientists a new way of attacking the cell to starve it, stop it from reproducing, and stop vessels from supplying nutrients to it. Simultaneously, modern medicine is opening to what they have denominated alternative treatments. More and more are being integrated into the modern war on cancer. These treatments include the use of nutrition and the mind.

Scientists are studying how the mind influences the body. This influence is not only in the subconscious mind but now in the conscious mind. How to eliminate stress from our lives through meditation is a good example. How with neurolinguistics, we can help our immune system function better. Huge scientific strides are being made in these fields.

So, our first step is to see cancer as a challenge, and not as something external that we cannot control. Once we do this, the mind thinks it as a problem to be solved. We focus on the solutions and not on the effects. This is huge, as it will change your paradigms, and you will see the huge possibility of beating the disease. Once you get to this stage, the next one is crucial. Now you must BELIEVE that you will beat this disease.

Listen to your internal voices. I say it in plural because we all have a positive voice and a negative voice. These voices are one of the collateral functions of the mind. They are more harmful than good. They bring doubt, indecision, and despair. We should use the mind as an instrument to solve problems, act, and maintain the body in harmony. These voices are just a byproduct of these processes. The enormous problem is that we forget who is in control. Is it you or is it your mind? These voices are not us; they are our minds trying to decipher situations based on prejudice, experience, adverse circumstances of the past, or teachings from our teachers, parents, mentors, and more. Yet what happens when we quiet our minds, and with it our voices? Nothing, on the contrary, it gives us clarity on the job at hand and to act. If we make the wrong choice? Well, we simply correct it and go on. The past is gone, and we do not know what the future has planned for us. So, live in your present and act on present situations.

Neurolinguistics is an important tool for the fight against cancer. We eradicate culpability, auto-compassion, procrastination, and despair. We analyze the situation for what it is. An adverse situation, like many more that we confront in our daily lives, that must be dealt with. A situation that we are going to beat.

One infallible way to feel this power is to take some time for yourself in a quiet place and think of five things you would like to forgive, including yourself. Say them aloud, and then think of ten reasons that you should be thankful for. However small they are but name them. The elation and peace that you will feel afterward will give you a clean slate in your spirit to conquer the universe. Just say to yourself: "I am going to win". This will become your war cry, and you will use it in difficult times and pleasant moments. It will take you throughout your treatment to a successful result.

THE STATE OF MIND

It was a little more difficult for me to listen to the doctor that I had cancer the second time. Yet, I did not give up. I was aware that I had to alter my approach and shift from being passive. I gave up control of my life and body, letting the doctors do their job. I went online and scoured books to gain a better understanding of my illness. Just as you are doing at this moment. What changed in me was my attitude. I was determined to fight this battle and emerge victorious.

I was not simply going through the motions of being a good patient and letting the doctors do their work. I had to take the initiative and be mindful of my environment, thoughts, and diet. All this did not interfere with the treatments, but that simply strengthen my spirit, my resolution, and my body.

This book is the result of the many hours I spent reading and informing myself about procedures and the success factors. It surprised me to see that mindset was one of the important differentiators of success and failure. Your state of mind is important, subconsciously it helps the body recover and fight the disease.

A note that is important to all patients. Pain can debilitate and bring depression. It will drain your will to fight. Please, talk to your doctor about it. Look for professional help and liberate yourself from this. Pain is not part of the side effects of treatment. Don't brave the pain. There is no prize at the end. It will only hinder your mind from focusing on getting better.

I have met doctors that believe that a positive state of mind will make a difference in the outcome. We must change our attitude towards the illness. We must transform ourselves into different people, a person who now sees life differently, and more importantly how we see ourselves.

In our quiet moments, thoughts will invade our minds. One recurring thought that kept on crawling in my mind was the question of how I got here. I would constantly reel back into my life and saw that it was chaos. As a TV executive, I thought that the more stress I had in my life, the more I accomplished. How stupid! But I honestly believed in it, to where if I had no stress, I would create it.

I started analyzing the past two years of my life, and it surprised me to see how stressed and depressed I was. I just wasn't conscious of it. I would hide in my work, which just fed my stress. So, what took me to this moment, to having cancer a second time? Well, a divorce, a change of job, and a change of country were important factors of stress and depression. These alone do not bring you cancer. Many factors cause cancer, as I have mentioned before. There is no direct link between cancer and stress. Yet I am convinced that this was the detonator in my case. It devastated my immune system, my nutrition was lousy, and my alcohol consumption was increasing. All because of stress and depression. My body just simply gave up, and as a result, my cancer appeared again.

So, we must make a conscious analysis of our lives. The levels of stress we are living, the type of nutrition we are consuming, and the environment we live in. Are our emotions under control? Do we express them healthily? Or do we just bottle them until there is an explosion? All these feelings contribute. We have to learn to handle them healthily and be able to express them peacefully. We must learn how to laugh, learn how to cry, learn how to love, and express gratitude.

My family, my friends, and my children were an enormous factor in helping me along. I let things be, eradicate judgment, and do not take myself so seriously. I killed my ego, and let my being come out. "Hello, this is who I am," I would say to the mirror. Then I would say to myself that whatever happened, I would confront it when it came and not before. I would just do my best and no more. And if the outcome was not the desired one, I would change the decision until I achieved the outcome. I understood that life is a constant struggle, yet if you change your attitude toward this struggle, it can be quite enjoyable. Celebrate all your successes as small as they may be, and face your failures, as you have now learned a new thing.

I can now say that thanks to cancer, I can evaluate every second of life with joy in my heart. I reflect on the incredible power my relationships have and thank them all for I love their laughter, their inspiration, their council, and the moments we share in silence.

Finally, I practice self-discipline. My discipline in my nutrition is to leave alcohol and tobacco, sugar, and processed food. To have a good night's sleep, to take my supplements, to meditate, and to be thankful for everything around me. To think that every problem that appears in my life is an opportunity. I do all this consciously, every day, and it gives me a sense of accomplishment that makes me feel good. It gives me well-being and life satisfaction.

Yes, I changed my life, and even if it sounds odd, I did it thanks to cancer. Now I live more consciously and take very few things for granted. I have learned that happiness is not outside me, it's inside. I have learned to forgive and to forgive myself. I have learned to live.

SUMMARY

CHANGE OF LIFE

Most people who have gone through this illness and endured the treatments of radiation and chemo take to a critical state of mind. They go through a total evaluation of their lives. This is normal, yet during treatment, patients should focus only on their recovery. They will have plenty of time to reflect on their way of life and what took them to their present situation.

When you analyze your levels of stress, quality of nutrition, exercise, and lifestyle, there is a good possibility that you realize that there must be a change.

THE POWER OF THE MIND

It is fundamental to recognize the power of our minds over our bodies. The importance lies in that we can use this power to influence our thoughts to the positive so that our bodies can act and change habits and ways of life.

VISUALIZATION

One technique that is used to make our minds more positive is using visualization. This technique comprises visualizing or imagining in our minds a desired outcome, and how it would feel to be in that position. We can include other senses in this technique, like taste, smell, and touch. It will help the mind communicate with the subconscious where we want to influence a positive outcome and eradicate all negative thoughts.

INTERNAL VOICE

We all have two voices in our minds. The positive and the negative. What we should try to do is to quiet the negative thoughts. We can do this by being conscious that they exist, and that we can control them. One way of helping this process is to use neurolinguistics. This technique uses repetition in our mind with a positive mantra: "I am going to win", "I am going to be healthy" and "I am going to beat this cancer". When we say it, and we think it over and over, even if there is a certain doubt, the subconscious takes it as a fact and helps the body to heal itself.

With a positive voice, we can have more energy, and we can change our attitude toward the disease and feel stronger to fight it.

MENTAL STATE

The attitude that transformed my way of looking at cancer was when I saw it as a challenge, "I am going to beat cancer".

I changed my bad habits, poor nutrition, exercise, and lifestyle. I lived in the present and let the past go. I got strong in discipline by just doing what was necessary and not thinking too much about what had to be done. Loving my family, my friends, and especially life.

CONCLUSION

We have seen how to prepare, go through treatments, nutrition, and have a good mind to beat cancer. I cannot say that it is easy, yet it is a fight that if you arrive at it with no knowledge, it can take you through a very tough path. 90% of the people I have talked to, that are in remission, say that they saw cancer as a challenge.

In 2004, they diagnosed me with cancer in the esophagus. I went through all the treatments the doctors told me to take as the protocols dictated. Chemo, radiation, and surgery. After that, I shook the doctor's hand and went back to my old lifestyle. The same stress, same diet, and strong desire to catch up with lost time.

In 2007, they diagnosed me with cancer again. I couldn't go back to the same treatments, in the same state of mind. What changed? I changed everything that I could control. I took control of my life and my diet. I studied what nourishments my body needed. Changed my mental attitude and my state of mind. I looked at ways of being more relaxed and more determined to fight. Exercised more and listened to my body. Was it easy? No. I had to eradicate my prejudices about diet, stress, and relaxing techniques, and to learn more about the power of the mind.

All the above I share so that you know what I did. Now the choice is yours.

I hope this book helps all those people that are suffering from cancer to understand that although this is a difficult disease, that can be beaten. With the correct attitude, excellent treatment, a conscientious diet, and a change of lifestyle will be the correct path.

In most cases that I interviewed, they would say that thanks to cancer they had found a true meaning of life, with a more sensitive view of themselves and their peers. They had found a new direction in their lives, putting the emphasis, on goodness, compassion, charity, and spiritual peace.

After all these years, when I ask myself, who am I? I can easily answer the question. I am a warrior.

A constant fighter against cancer. After 15 years, I still fight against it. I know it is there in my body, but now I am in control. I will keep this in control till the end of my days. I listen more to my body; I try to keep all in balance, for that is the homeostasis of life, and thank the universe that I had the chance to travel this road and wake up to reality.

Now it is my turn to share it.

I invite you to become a conscious warrior, with your mind and body, you fight off the molecular attack our body is going through. To love life with all your heart, knowing that it will constantly send you messages about its existence, and embrace the challenge.

With all my heart, I wish you the best in your journey.

Lawrence W. Dickins

cancerfighttowin@gmail.com

GLOSSARY

Adaptogen A balancing nontoxic plant extract, with properties to promote balance of substances in the body, increase the body's ability to resist the damaging effects of stress, and promote or restore normal physiological functioning.

Algologist A doctor specializing in the study and treatment of pain.

Amino acids. These are substances containing nitrogen and hydrogen and which are found in proteins.

Anaerobic. Living, active, occurring, or existing in the absence of free oxygen. As opposed to aerobic which means, living, active, occurring, or existing in the presence of oxygen.

Anastomosis. It is a surgical connection between two structures. It usually means a connection that is created between tubular structures such as blood vessels, loops of the intestine, etc.

Angiogenesis. The development of new blood vessels.

Anti-exudative. A substance that prevents a fluid rich in protein and cellular elements from oozing out of the blood vessels due to inflammation and deposited in nearby tissues.

Antigen. A harmful substance that enters the body which causes the body to make antibodies as a response to fight disease. For example, a common cold virus.

Antineoplastic. Acting to prevent, inhibit or halt the development of neoplasm or tumor.

Antioxidants. A substance that removes toxins from your body and protects against harmful molecules like free radicals.

Antiseptic. An antimicrobial substance that is applied to living tissue to reduce the possibility of infection, sepsis, or putrefaction.

Apigenin. A substance found in many plants that is a natural product belonging to the flavones class and existing as a glycoside.

Apoptosis. Is a form of programmed cell death that occurs in multicellular organisms.

Aromatase inhibitor. A drug that inhibits the enzyme aromatase and a means of lowering the level of estrogen estradiol.

Atypical Ductal Hyperplasia (ADH), found in 5% to 20% of breast biopsies, is a high-risk precursor lesion. While not carcinoma, it has the potential to progress to DCIS or invasive carcinoma.

Atypical Lobular Hyperplasia (ALH) is a non-cancerous breast lesion with abnormal cell growth in the lobules. It indicates a slightly increased risk of future breast cancer in the same breast. Regular monitoring or further evaluation may be advised.

Benign. Of a mild type or character that does not threaten health or life especially not becoming cancerous.

Beta-carotene. A reddish-orange pigment that is an isomer of carotene found chiefly in orange, dark green, and yellow vegetables and fruits, that is converted into vitamin A in the body.

Biopsy. The removal of a sample of tissue for examination under a microscope to check for cancer cells or other abnormalities.

Blanching. A cooking process wherein a food, usually a vegetable or fruit, is scalded in boiling water, removed after a brief, timed interval, and finally plunged into ice-cold water, to halt the cooking process.

BRCA GENES are genes that produce proteins that help repair damaged DNA. Everyone has two copies of each of these genes—one copy inherited from each parent.

Bronchial epithelium. It is a key element of the respiratory airways. It constitutes the interface between the environment and the host. It is a physical barrier with many chemical and immunological properties.

Cancer grade. A system for classifying cancer cells in terms of how abnormal they appear when examined under a microscope. The objective is to provide information about the probable growth rate of the tumor and its tendency to spread. The system varies with each type of tumor.

Capsaicin. It is an active component of chili peppers that gives its hot taste and is used to relieve muscle pain, joint pain, and nerve pain associated with osteoarthritis, rheumatoid arthritis, and diabetic neuropathy.

Carcinoma. It is a type of cancer that in cells that start that make up the skin or the tissue lining the organs such as the liver or kidneys.

Carnosol. Is a phenolic diterpene found in the herbs Rosemary and Mountain desert sage. It has been studied in-vitro for anti-cancer effects in various cancer cell types.

Catechins. Polyphenolic flavanol catechins in green tea have antiviral, antioxidant, and chemopreventive properties. The most potent is epigallocatechin-3-gallate EGCG.

Catheter. A flexible tube that is inserted through a narrow opening into a body cavity, as in the bladder to remove the fluid.

Chemotherapy Cycles A course of treatment that is repeated in regular intervals with periods of rest in between. For example, treatment given for one week followed by three weeks of rest is one treatment cycle.

Chemotherapy. Is the use of drugs to treat any disease. The most common use is in drugs used in cancer treatment acting in cells throughout the body.

Cholesterol. It's a type of fat found in the blood. The liver makes cholesterol for your body. Cholesterol is also found in food. The two main types are: LDL (low-density lipoprotein) which is considered the bad cholesterol as it tends to stick to the blood vessels. HDL (high-density lipoprotein) is considered the good cholesterol which carries the cholesterol in the blood back to the liver where is broken down.

Circulating Tumor Cells (CTCs) are cancer cells that split away from the primary tumor and appear in the circulatory system as singular units or clusters,

Cytokines. They are broad and lose kinds of small proteins that are important in cell signaling. Their release influences the behavior of cells around them.

Daidzein. A phytoestrogen plant molecule that is structurally and functionally like mammalian estrogens. It is found in soybeans.

Diuretic. A substance that increases the passage of urine.

DNA. Deoxyribonucleic acid is a molecule composed of two chains that coil around each other to form a double helix carrying the genetic instructions used in the growth, development functioning, and reproduction of all known living organisms.

Ductal carcinoma in situ (DCIS) is when breast milk duct cells become cancerous but haven't spread to surrounding tissue. It's a non-invasive form of breast cancer.

Echinacea is a genus of herbaceous flowering. They are traditionally used to boost the immune system.

Ellagic Acid. It is a natural phenol antioxidant compound found in strawberries, raspberries, blackberries, cherries, and walnuts. It is known for its anti-cancer properties.

Endoscopy is a procedure used in medicine to look inside the body. It uses an endoscope, a flexible tube with a light and camera attached to it, which is inserted into the cavities of the body.

Estrogen. It is the primary female sex hormone. It is responsible for the development and regulation of the female reproductive system and secondary sex characteristics. Three major endogenous estrogens in females have activity: Estrone, estradiol, and estriol.

Exogenic Nutrients. They are nutrients that are found outside the body and that are ingested and broken down into simple chemical compounds for their absorption.

FDA. The Food and Drug Administration is a federal agency of the United States Department of Health and Human

Services that regulate and protect the use of some food, cosmetic, and drugs

Fibroadenoma is the most common type of benign breast tumor, and most don't increase your risk of breast cancer. Although women of any age can develop fibroadenomas, they usually occur in younger, premenopausal women.

Fibrocystic breasts are lumpy or ropelike in texture due to nodular or glandular breast tissue. It's common to have fibrocystic breasts or experience changes in them, but it's not a disease. These fluctuations in breast texture with the menstrual cycle are considered normal. Medical professionals now use the terms "fibrocystic breasts" or "fibrocystic breast changes" instead of "fibrocystic breast disease."

Flavonoids. They are a variety of phytonutrients (plant chemicals) found in almost all fruits and vegetables. Along with carotenoids they are responsible for the vivid colors of fruits and vegetables. They are powerful antioxidants with anti-inflammatory and immune system benefits.

Free Radicals. They are unstable atoms that can damage cells, causing illness and aging.

Genistein. It is a phytoestrogen that is described as an angiogenesis (blood vessel growth) inhibitor. It is found in soybeans.

Glucans. Beta-glucans are sugars that are found in the cell walls of bacteria. Fungi, algae, lichens, and plants, such as oats and barley. They are used for fighting high cholesterol, diabetes, HIV/AIDS, and cancer.

Glycitein. It is also a phytoestrogen with a weak estrogenic activity compared to the other soy isoflavones.

HER2-positive Breast Cancer is a type of aggressive breast cancer with too much HER2 protein. It affects about 20% of breast cancer cases. Targeted therapies have improved treatment outcomes.

Hormones are regulatory substances produced in an organism and transported in tissue fluids such as blood or sap to stimulate specific cells or tissues into action.

Hyperplasia. It is the enlargement of an organ or tissue that results from cell proliferation. It may lead to gross enlargement of an organ, and the term is sometimes confused with benign neoplasia or benign tumor.

Invasive ductal carcinoma (IDC) is a form of breast cancer that originates in the milk ducts and can spread to nearby tissues and beyond through lymph nodes or the bloodstream.

Isoflavones. They are phytochemicals, that are found in plants. They are also a type of phytoestrogen, or plant hormone, that resembles human estrogen in chemical structure, yet they are weaker.

Kupffer Cells. They are large and specialized cells, macrophages that defend the body from pathogens and are found in the liver.

Letininan. It is a beta-glucan found in Shitake mushrooms found to help with cancer.

Leukemia. Cancer of the blood cells is caused by a rise in the number of white blood cells in the body.

Leukocyte. It is a white blood cell. A colorless cell that circulates in the blood and body fluids and is involved in counteracting foreign substances and disease.

Lycopene. It is a bright red carotene and carotenoid pigment and phytochemical found in tomatoes and other red fruit and vegetables, such as red carrots, watermelons, and papaya. It is a powerful antioxidant that lowers the risk of cancer.

Macronutrients. They are substances that are required in large amounts by living organisms. Fats, proteins, and carbohydrates are examples.

Mastocytes. It is a white blood cell, containing many granules rich in histamine and heparin.

Metaplasia. It is the transformation of one differentiated cell type to another differentiated cell type. The change may be part of a normal maturation process or caused by some sort of abnormal stimulus.

Metastasis. It is the spreading of cancer from its point of origin to other parts of the body.

Minerals. They are chemical substances the body needs as building units.

Mitosis. It is the ordinary division of a body cell (somatic cell) to form two daughter cells, each with the same chromosomes as the parent cell.

Monoclonal Antibodies. (mAb or moAb) These are antibodies that are made by identical immune cells that are all clones of a unique parent cell. They are used in immunotherapy processes.

Mouth Sores. Mouth Ulcers or Mucositis are caused many times as a side effect of chemotherapy or radiation treatment. This is because the drugs used, or the radiation kill fast-growing cells in the mouth's lining.

MRI. It is a Magnetic Resonance Imaging that is used in diagnostic techniques, using magnetic fields and radio waves to produce detailed imaging of the body's soft tissue and bones.

Myalgia. It is the pain in a muscle or group of muscles.

Nausea. It is the feeling of sickness with an inclination to vomit. This can be caused by the treatments of chemotherapy and radiation.

Neurolinguistics. It is the branch of linguistics dealing with the relationship between language and the structure and functioning of the brain.

Neutrophils. They are a common type of white blood cells important in fighting off infections, particularly those caused by bacteria.

Nitrosamines. A type of chemical found in tobacco products and tobacco smoke, Nitrosamines are also found in many fried foods and meat. Some nitrosamines increase the risk of cancer.

Oncologist surgeon. He is a surgeon who specialized in the biopsy and removal of tumors.

Oncologist. He is a doctor who specialized in the diagnosis and treatment of cancer.

Orchiectomy. It is a surgical procedure in which one or both testicles are removed.

Papilloma is a benign (non-cancerous) tumor arising from an epithelial surface and usually known to grow in an outward direction.

Pathogen. It is a bacterium, virus, or other microorganism that can cause disease.

PET Scan. Positron Emission Tomography is a nuclear medicine functional imaging technique that is used to observe metabolic processes in the body as an aid to the diagnosis of diseases including cancer.

Phagocytes. It is a type of cell that can engulf, ingest and digest foreign particles, such as bacteria, carbon, or dyes, and form part of the immune system.

Phytochemicals. They are chemicals found in plants.

Polyphenols. These form part of a large group of phytochemicals which are naturally occurring micronutrients in plants. These compounds give a plant its color and can help them protect them from various dangers.

Polysaccharide. It is a large molecule made of many smaller monosaccharides such as glucose, fructose, and galactose.

Three important polysaccharides are starch, glycogen, and cellulose.

Portable infusion pump. It is a medical device used externally to deliver fluids into a patient's body in a controlled manner.

Processed Foods. Any food item that has had a series of mechanical or chemical operations performed on it to change or preserve it. These are usually those foods that come in a box or a bag and contain more than one item on the list of ingredients.

Pruritus. It is the severe itching of the skin as a symptom of various ailments

Radiologists These are doctors that specialize in diagnosing and treating injuries and diseases using medical imaging procedures such as X-rays, computed tomography, magnetic resonance imaging, nuclear medicine, positron emission tomography, and ultrasound.

Sarcoma. A type of cancer that starts in the bone or other soft tissue of the body including cartilage, fat, muscle, and blood vessels. Fibrous tissue, or other connective or supportive tissue. Different types of sarcoma are based on where the cancer forms. For example, osteosarcoma, forms in the bones, liposarcoma, forms in fatty tissue, and rhabdomyosarcoma forms in muscle.

Stage. Staging helps to determine where cancer is located, if or where it has spread, and whether it is affecting other parts of the body.

Sulphurafane. It is a chemical that is found in certain types of vegetables such as broccoli, cabbage, and cauliflower. It helps in the prevention of prostate cancer, and other types of cancer.

Terpenes. They are aromatic organic compounds found in many plants. They are developed to ward off herbivores that might eat them, and attract helpful predators, and pollinators. Cannabis has naturally high levels of terpenes.

Testosterone. A "male" hormone produced by the testes that encourage the development of male sexual characteristics. The ovaries and adrenal cortex also produce this hormone.

The Immune System is made up of special cells, proteins, tissues, and organs that protect the host from environmental agents such as microbes or chemicals, thereby preserving the integrity of the body.

Tomography. A method of producing a 3D image of the internal structures of a solid object such as a human body, by the observation and recording of the differences in the effects of passaging waves of energy in those structures.

Triple-Negative Breast Cancer (TNBC) is a type of aggressive breast cancer that lacks three specific receptors: estrogen receptor, progesterone receptor, and HER2 protein. It comprises about 10-15% of breast cancer cases and mainly affects younger women with limited treatment options. Chemotherapy is the primary treatment for TNBC.

Tumor Markers. It is a biomarker found in the blood, urine, and body tissue that can be elevated by one or more types of cancers. There are many types of tumor markers, each indicative of a specific type of disease process, and they are used in oncology to help detect the presence of cancer.

Tumor. A swelling of a part of the body usually with no inflammation, is caused by an abnormal multiplication of cells and growth of tissue whether benign or malignant.

Ultrasound. It is the imaging through high-frequency sound waves. Ultrasound waves can be bounced off tissues by using special devices. The echoes are then converted into pictures called sonograms.

Vaccine. It is a substance used to stimulate the production of antibodies and provide immunity against one or several diseases. They are prepared from the causative agent of a disease, its product, or a synthetic substitute, treated to act as an antigen without inducing the disease.

Visualization. It is a cognitive tool accessing imagination to realize all aspects of an object, action, or outcome. This may include recreating a mental sensory experience of sound, sight, smell, taste, and touch.

Vitamin. Any or various organic substances that are essential in minute quantities to the nutrition of most animals and some plants. Vitamins do not provide energy or serve as building units but are essential in regulating metabolic processes.

CANCER SUPPORT

USA

Breast Cancer.org

https://www.breastcancer.org/treatment/complementary-therapy/types/support-groups

American Cancer Society. Support and Online Communities.Telephone:800.227.2345 https://www.cancer.org/

Cancer Care. https://www.cancercare.org/support_groups/

City of Hope. Telephone: 800-826-4673

Cancer.Net www.cancer.net/support/

National Cancer Institute. List of 106 support groups throughout the USA. Telephone 1-800-4-CANCER https://supportorgs.cancer.gov/

CANADA

Canadian Breast Cancer Network

https://cbcn.ca/en/support_groups

Canadian Cancer Society. https://cancer.ca/en/living-with-cancer/how-we-can-help

Toronto Central Health Line.
https://www.torontocentralhealthline.ca/

Type Cancer Support Groups in the search box.

Quebec Cancer Foundation.
https://fqc.qc.ca/en

UNITED KINGDOM

Breast Cancer Support UK.
https://breastcancersupport.org.uk/

Cancer Support UK.
https://cancersupportuk.org/

Macmillan Cancer Support.
https://community.macmillan.org.uk/

Additionally, most Hospitals in these countries have their own Support Group, or they can guide you to one.

REFERENCES

[i] Bassil KL, Vakil C, Sanborn M, Cole D C, Kaur J S, Kerr K J. "Cancer health effects of pesticides: systematic review" Can Fam Physician 2007 Oct; 53(10):1704-11. https://pubmed.ncbi.nlm.nih.gov/17934034/

[ii] "Psychological Stress and Cancer" was originally published by The National Cancer Institute in Dec.10, 2012. https://www.cancer.gov/about-cancer/coping/feelings/stress-fact-sheet

[iii] Zivkovic I., Rakin A., Petrovic-Djergovic D. Miljkovic B., Micic M. "The effects of chronic stress on thymus innervation in the adult rat" Acta Histochemical Vol.106, Issue 6, Feb. 24, 2205 Pgs. 449-458 https://doi.org/10.1016/j.acthis.2004.11.002

[iv] American Cancer Society. Cancer Facts & Figures 2020. Atlanta: American Cancer Society; 2020. https://www.cancer.org/content/dam/cancer-org/research/cancer-facts-and-statistics/annual-cancer-facts-and-figures/2020/cancer-facts-and-figures-2020.pdf

[v] Cristol H. "Exercise Linked with Lower Risk of 13 Types of Cancer" American Cancer Society Atlanta: American Cancer Society 2016. https://www.cancer.org/latest-news/exercise-linked-with-lower-risk-of-13-types-of-cancer.html

[vi] Rahner N, Steinke V. Hereditary Cancer Syndromes. Deutsches Arzteblatt International Oct, 2008 Dtsch Arztebl Int. 2008 Oct; 105(41):706-14 doi: 10.3238/arztebl.2008.0706. National Library of Medicine PubliMed Central 2008. https://pubmed.ncbi.nlm.nih.gov/19623293/

[vii] Tian, L., Xu, B., Chen, Y. *et al.* Specific targeting of glioblastoma

with an oncolytic virus expressing a cetuximab-CCL5 fusion protein via innate and adaptive immunity. *Nat Cancer* **3**, 1318–1335 (2022). https://doi.org/10.1038/s43018-022-00448-0

viii Yan Cui, Thomas E Rohan "Vitamin D, calcium, and breast cancer risk: a review" National Library of Medicine August 10, 2006. doi: 10.1158/1055-9965.EPI-06-0075. PMID: 16896028 https://pubmed.ncbi.nlm.nih.gov/16896028/#:~:text=Vitamin%20D%20and%20calcium%20are,normal%20and%20malignant%20breast%20cells.

ix Vodnala SK, Eil R, Restifo NP, et al. T cell stemness and dysfunction in tumors are triggered by a common mechanism. Science. March 29, 2019. DOI: 10.1126/science.aau0135 https://www.cancer.gov/news-events/press-releases/2019/stemness-potassium-immunotherapy#:~:text=Dying%20cancer%20cells%20release%20the,to%20eliminate%20cancer%20during%20immunotherapy.

x Medically reviewed by Christina Chun, MPH — By Alex Snyder — Updated on September 18, 2018. "How selenium helps Protect against Cancer" Healthline https://www.healthline.com/health/anti-cancer-supplements

xi Guang-Jian Du, Zhiyu Zhang, Xiao-Dong Wen, Chunhao Yu, Tyler Calway, Chun-Su Yuan, and Chong-Zhi Wang "Epigallocatechin Gallate (EGCG) Is the Most Effective Cancer Chemopreventive Polyphenol in Green Tea" published in National Library of Medicine 2012 Nov 8 doi: 10.3390/nu4111679 https://www.ncbi.nlm.nih.gov/pmc/articles/PMC3509513/

xii Zhou DH, Wang X, Yang M, Shi X, Huang W, Feng Q. Combination of low concentration of (-)-epigallocatechin gallate (EGCG) and curcumin strongly suppresses the growth of non-small cell lung cancer in vitro and in vivo through causing cell cycle arrest. Int J Mol Sci. 2013 Jun 5;14(6):12023-36. doi: 10.3390/ijms140612023. PMID: 23739680; PMCID: PMC3709771. https://www.ncbi.nlm.nih.gov/pmc/articles/PMC3709771/

xiii Y. Shukla, M. Singh "Cancer Preventive properties of ginger; a Brief review" Environmental Carcinogenesis Division, Industrial Toxicology Research Center, Uttar Pradesh, India. July 2006.

www.sciencedirect.com

xiv . "Spices for Prevention and treatment of cancer. J. Zheng, Y Zhou, Hua-Bin Li School of Public Health, Sun Yat-sen University Guangzhou China. ncbi.nim.nih.gov

xv National Cancer Institute "Cruciferous Vegetables and Cancer Prevention" 7 June 2012. www.cancer.gov

xvi Johnson E.J. "The role of carotenoids in human health" 2002 http//pubmed.ncbi.nlm.nih.gov

xvii Nancy E Moran, Jennifer M Thomas-Ahner, Lei Wan, Krystle E Zuniga, John W Erdman, Jr, Steven K Clinton, Tomatoes, Lycopene, and Prostate Cancer: What Have We Learned from Experimental Models?, *The Journal of Nutrition*, Volume 152, Issue 6, June 2022, Pages 1381–1403, https://doi.org/10.1093/jn/nxac066.

xviii Physicians Committee, for responsible medicine "How Soy Isoflavones Help Protect Against Cancer" www.pcrm.org.

xix Chikov N. Chikov N. "Six cancer–Fighting Medicinal Mushrooms, Dr. Nalini Chikov in 2012 and updated in December 2017 HuffPost The Blog Anticancer living. https://www.huffpost.com/entry/cancer-foods_b_1192207

xx Patel S. and Goyal A. "Recent developments in mushrooms as anti-cancer therapeutics: a review" Seema Patel and Arum Goyal. NHI Nov 25 2011doi: 10.1007/s13205-011-0036-2. https://pubmed.ncbi.nlm.nih.gov/22582152/

xxi Yang Y., Ikezoe T., Zheng Z., Taguchi H., Koeffler P. and Zhu W.G. "Saw Palmetto induces growth arrest and apoptosis of androgen-dependent prostate cancer LNCaP cells via inactivation of STAT 3 and androgen receptor signaling" Pub Med Gov. Sep 31, 2007. 1 Department of Biochemistry and Molecular Biology, Peking University Health Science Center, Beijing 100083, P.R. China; 2Department of Hematology and Respiratory Medicine, Kochi Medical School, Kochi University, Okohcho, Nankoku, Kochi 783-8505, Japan; 3Division of Hematology and Oncology, June 21, 2007, International Journal of Oncology 31: 593/600 2007.

file:///C:/Users/numar/Downloads/ijo_31_3_593_PDF%20(2).pdf
https://pubmed.ncbi.nlm.nih.gov/17671686/

xxii . Pretner W.E. Amri H., Li W, Brown R., Lin C.S., Makarou E.,
Defeudis F.V., Drieu K.,Papadopoulos V., "Cancer-relate
overexpression of the peripheral-type" Jan-Feb 26 National
Library of Medicine https://pubmed.ncbi.nlm.nih.gov/16475673/

xxiii Chao, JC; Chu, CC. Effects of Gingko Biloba extract on cell
proliferation and cytotoxicity in human hepatocellular carcinoma
cells. World J Gastroenterol.2004 Jan 10 (1): 37-41.) National
Library of Medicine: https://doi.org/10.3748/wjg.v10.i1.37

xxiv Kotakadi V.S., Yu Jin, Holseth A.B. et all. "Ginkgo biloba extract
EGb 761 has anti-inflammatory properties and ameliorates colitis
in mice by driving effector T cell apoptosis" September 2008
National Library of Medicine, Carcinogenesis. National Library of
Medicine: https://doi.org/10.1093%2Fcarcin%2Fbgn143

xxv Jung Da, Mingxi Xu, Yiwei Wang, Wenfeng Li, M ujun Lu Zhong
Wang. "Kaempferol Promotes Apoptosis While Inhibiting Cell
Proliferation Via Androgen-Dependent Pathway and suppressing
Vasculogenic Mimicry and Invasion in Prostate Cancer"
Analytical Cellular Pathology 2019: 1907698 published online
National Library of Medicine:
https://doi.org/10.1155/2019/1907698

xxvi Kwang-Soo Baek, Young-Su Yi; Jae, Young-Jin Son, Deok Jeong,
Nak Yoon Sung, Aditha Aravinthan, Jong-Hoon Kim, Jae Youl
Cho. "Comparison of anticancer activities of Korean Red
Ginseng-derived fractions." 2017 Jul. National Library of
Medicine: https://doi.org/10.1016/j.jgr.2016.11.001

xxvii Dangor J. "Ginseng fights fatigue in cancer patients" Mayo Clinic
Newsletter May 31, 2012. Published www.mayo.edu,
https://newsnetwork.mayoclinic.org/discussion/ginseng-fights-
fatigue-in-cancer-patients-mayo-clinic-led-study-finds/

xxviii Chao-Yan Wu; Yuan Ke; Yi-Frei Zeng Ying-Wen Zhang; Hai-Jun
Yu "Anticancer activity of Astralagus polysaccharide in human
non-small cell lung cancer cells". PubMed.gov Cancer cell Int.

2017 Dec 4; PMID 29225515. PMCID PMC 5716001 DOI: 10.1186/s12935-017-6 2017 published in the National Library of Medicine https://doi.org/10.1186%2Fs12935-017-0487-6

xxix Hussain A.: Sharma C.; Khan S.; Shah K.; Haque S. "Aloe vera inhibits proliferation of human breast cancer and cervical cancer cells and acts synergistically with cisplatin" PMID: 25854386 DOI 10.7314/apjcp.2015 16.7.29390 Published in PubMed gov 2015. From: https://doi.org/10.7314/apjcp.2015.16.7.2939

xxx Stoller R. "Cancer-Fighting Cocoa" August 15,2016. Blog. Cancer Fighting Food, Cancer Fighting Lifestyle at NFCR Blog | Cancer–Fighting Cocoa - National Foundation for Cancer Research (nfcr.org) https://newsnetwork.mayoclinic.org/discussion/ginseng-fights-fatigue-in-cancer-patients-mayo-clinic-led-study-finds/

xxxi Ramirez JK., Guarner F., BustosL., Maruy A., Sdepanian V., Cohen H. "Antibiotics as Major Disruptors of Gut Microbiota" Published online 2020 Nov 24 National Library of Medicine https://doi.org/10.3389/fcimb.2020.572912

xxxii Ciernikova S., Mego M.,Chovanec M. "Exploring the Potential Role of the Gut Microbiome in Chemotherapy-Induced Neurocognitive Disorders and Cardiovascular Toxicity" Published online 2021 Feb 13. National Library of Medicine https://doi.org/10.3390/cancers13040782

Made in the USA
Monee, IL
02 October 2024